STANLEY SAMUEL HARAKAS is Archbishop Iakovos Professor of Orthodox Theology at Holy Cross Greek Orthodox School of Theology. Among his recent works are *Contemporary Moral Issues Facing the Orthodox Christian, Let Mercy Abound: A Chronicle of Greek Orthodox Social Concerns*, and *Toward Transfigured Life: The Theoria of Eastern Orthodox Ethics.*

Health and Medicine
in the Eastern Orthodox
Tradition

Health/Medicine and the Faith Traditions

Edited by James P. Wind

Health/Medicine and the Faith Traditions
explores the ways in which major religions
relate to the questions of human well-being.
It issues from Project Ten, an interfaith program
of The Park Ridge Center for the Study of
Health, Faith, and Ethics.

Barbara Hofmaier, Publications Coordinator

The Park Ridge Center
is part of the Lutheran General Health Care System.

The Park Ridge Center
676 N. St. Clair, Suite 450
Chicago, Illinois 60611

Health
and Medicine in the
Eastern Orthodox
Tradition

Faith, Liturgy, and Wholeness

Stanley Samuel Harakas

Crossroad • New York

1990

The Crossroad Publishing Company
370 Lexington Avenue, New York, N.Y. 10017

Printed in the United States of America

Library of Congress Cataloging-in-Publication Data

Harakas, Stanley S.
    Health and medicine in the Eastern Orthodox tradition : faith, liturgy,
and wholeness / by Stanley Samuel Harakas.
        p.   cm.—(Health/medicine and the faith traditions)
    Includes index.
    ISBN 0-8245-0934-X
    1. Health—Religious aspects—Orthodox Eastern Church.
    2. Medicine—Religious aspects—Orthodox Eastern Church.
    3. Orthodox Eastern Church—Doctrines.   4. Orthodox Eastern Church-
-Liturgy. I. Title. II. Series.
BX323.H35   1990
261.8'321—dc20   89-9998
                                                                              CIP

To the only God, our Savior through
Jesus Christ our Lord, be glory, majesty,
dominion, and authority, before all time and
now and for ever. Amen. (Jude 25)

and

to the faithful parishioners of
Annunciation Greek Orthodox Church,
Newburyport, Massachusetts,
who know how to heal
in the Spirit of the Lord,
with gratitude.

Health/Medicine and the Faith Traditions

HEALTH AND MEDICINE IN THE ANGLICAN TRADITION
David H. Smith

HEALTH AND MEDICINE IN THE CATHOLIC TRADITION
Richard A. McCormick

HEALTH AND MEDICINE IN THE CHRISTIAN SCIENCE TRADITION
Robert Peel

HEALTH AND MEDICINE IN THE EASTERN ORTHODOX TRADITION
Stanley Samuel Harakas

HEALTH AND MEDICINE IN THE HINDU TRADITION
Prakash N. Desai

HEALTH AND MEDICINE IN THE ISLAMIC TRADITION
Fazlur Rahman

HEALTH AND MEDICINE IN THE JEWISH TRADITION
David M. Feldman

HEALTH AND MEDICINE IN THE LUTHERAN TRADITION
Martin E. Marty

HEALTH AND MEDICINE IN THE METHODIST TRADITION
E. Brooks Holifield

HEALTH AND MEDICINE IN THE REFORMED TRADITION
Kenneth L. Vaux

Contents

Foreword

Millions of Americans and hundreds of millions of world citizens cling to Orthodox traditions of faith and are members of Orthodox Christian churches. Those who tend the traditions and care for people who live by them will recognize Stanley Samuel Harakas as a reliable guide through the maze of teachings and practices having to do with health and wholeness. A well-respected theologian and ethicist, he has done as much as anyone in our generation to interpret Orthodoxy to its adherents and to explain it to other citizens. In this work he moves beyond his general interest in ethics to present what we believe to be the first comprehensive work on Orthodoxy in the context of health and modern medicine.

The book, like the other books in this series, has two purposes. For believers within the tradition it is a well of resources and a mirror for self-description. To others it is an important stream flowing by, with which they should be acquainted, as well as a window for learning about neighbors. In pluralist America where, as Father Harakas notes in line one, "the vast majority of Americans have little or no knowledge of the Eastern Orthodox Christian church," there is urgent need for such a work. The Orthodox are physicians and nurses and researchers; they are patients and supporters and seekers after wholeness. They play an overlooked but major part in the economy of medicine and spirituality.

The Western religionist who looks through this window will experience some shock of nonrecognition as a spiritual landscape first comes into view. The terms are similar to those one hears in Judaism, Catholicism, and Protestantism. Yet they connect with meanings which differ from those Western Europeans and their heirs around the world associate with these words and concepts.

Even the dedication page alerts us to the scope of Orthodox concern. On one hand it reaches to the New Testament and the formal liturgy for a passage of noble ascription to "the only God," showing something of the transcendental reach of this faith that would not be earthbound. But the author continues with a down-to-earth reference, a tender and pastoral address to a congregation "down the block," as it were. There, presumably, the people think of "the only God," but they also live full, rich, distracted lives, with signals about health and medicine coming their way from many sources, few of them Orthodox. For them, this book will afford a rediscovery of meanings, and maybe even a discovery. The feet-on-the-ground Westerner, familiar with books dedicated to a teacher, a relative, a friend, will face Harakas's recognition of a debt too large for such dedication-page lines. He must immediately move above and beyond to "the only God."

Each time I study another manuscript in this series I am forced to ask: what is distinctive about this tradition? In all cases there can be overlap between heritages, since so many books deal with heirs of the faith of Israel, also as embodied in a new covenant in Jesus Christ. So it is with the Roman Catholic, Anglican, Lutheran, Methodist, and similar traditions. They all have much in common. And yet how different they are from each other.

Let me take the most obvious example. Many Jews, Catholics, and Protestants, along with adherents of some other faiths, are familiar with the notion that in certain religious communities how one *acts* is the measure of faith. Others, such as ultraconservative Protestants and Catholics, recognize themselves in communities where *dogma* or doctrine helps constitute the foundation. In Orthodoxy, it is manifest from this book, the *liturgy*, the "people's service," the public act of worship is the source, the measure, the life-giver to all the parts.

The first time I read this manuscript I found that, following his helpful general introduction, the author took up liturgy and stayed with it. When, I asked myself, will he concentrate on the history of doctrine, since Orthodoxy cherishes true teaching (-*doxy*)? When will he come to the works of justice and love that are such a part of religion, of Christianity? Orthodoxy does cherish these, as the book makes clear. Then it occurred to me: Harakas *is* talking about the teaching of Orthodoxy, about the action within it, whenever he takes up liturgy in detail.

As this realization dawns upon readers, they are likely to become more patient with the accent on liturgy and then to see their patience grow to fascination. The book helps familiarize them with the heart of Orthodoxy and its aspirations to heal; it can help them refract the light of Orthodoxy into their own often quite different faith traditions and learn from what it shows. Since all religious communities engage in worship, one might ask: while the believers give glory to "the only God," are they also getting out of their liturgical acts, even if made up of humble forms of prayer and silent worship, all that they might for the care of their bodies and cure of their souls?

A fundamental reorientation occurs for the non-Orthodox just as a confirmation occurs here for the Orthodox. The visitor to the tradition learns to look at his or her own heritage in a new way. Let me illustrate with an example spanning an East-West boundary more distant than that drawn within Christianity between Orthodoxy and Western-based traditions. My colleague Anthony Yu spent years translating what became a four-volume publication, *The Journey to the West*. It is a centuries-old work of Chinese literature about a Buddhist monk and a monkey, an epic of sorts which fuses the sacred and the secular, the profoundly humanistic with the picaresque, the humorous, and the trivial in novel ways. Thinking I would show my at-homeness after having read two of the volumes, I said: "Tony, *now* I get it. *The Journey to the West* is the *Don Quixote* of the East." "No, you don't get it," he said in smiling reply; "*Don Quixote* is *The Journey to the West* of the West." He implied nothing arrogant, as his smile made clear; he suggested instead something perspectival, reorienting.

So it is, closer to home, with the mirrors and windows, the sources and streams, that meet each other in this book. Westerners may find themselves noting the ways in which, say, St. John Chrysostom is the Augustine of the East, when they might well be learning that St. Augustine is a Chrysostom of the West. Certainly they will come to terms with differing views of time and space. Stanley Harakas shows how he thinks of Chrysostom and Basil and others of long ago as his contemporaries, available here and now. And that thinking changes how one treats the acts that move a person through history and tradition: being born, suffering, dying.

The word *wholeness* appears in the subtitle of this book, as well it should. The term sometimes acquires faddish connotations in this new age of New Age thinking, but in these times when Westerners are learning from Buddhism and Hinduism or Christians are recovering elements of wholeness from Judaism, this word speaks directly to the center of Orthodoxy's vision and aspiration. It belongs here, offering riches to those in the tradition and beckoning those who must cross bridges to it.

Health and Medicine in the Eastern Orthodox Tradition is an exposition of this liturgical vision of wholeness by a lifelong inhabitant of the tradition and a major scholar. Between the transcendental grandeur of the first part of the dedication to this book and the communal warmth implied by the second part is where the Orthodox live and where they pursue wholeness.

Harakas helps situate them at the juncture and invites others to learn and profit from their sojourn in that situation.

Martin E. Marty

Part I

INTRODUCTION TO THE ORTHODOX CHURCH AND PEOPLE

· 1 ·

Tradition and History

The vast majority of Americans have little or no knowledge of the Eastern Orthodox Christian church. Yet as an organized body of believers it is one of the largest of the Christian churches. The reason for this paradox is that Americans trace the main sources of their identity to relatively recent Western European cultural traditions, while Orthodox Christianity is deeply rooted historically in Eastern Europe and the Near East. Until recently, little contact existed between Western Christendom and its counterpart in the East. Further, since about the year 1204 (and perhaps two centuries earlier) Western Christianity and Eastern Christianity were separated from each other by differences in doctrine, worship, governance, practice, mind-set, and culture. This was true despite their shared commitment to the Christian faith.

One purpose of this book is to help health care professionals (who themselves come from various religious traditions, or perhaps from none) to understand how the Orthodox Christian faith is related to issues of health and medicine so that they can serve their Orthodox patients with greater sensitivity. The book is also written to help Orthodox people understand more fully the relation of their tradition to the issues of health and medicine, as well as for those with a general interest in this formative Christian tradition. Because Orthodox Christianity will not be very familiar to the majority of the readers of this volume, it may be helpful to begin with an overview.[1]

As we begin, we should be aware that we are dealing here with a church that understands its history to be essentially identical with the two-thousand-year history of Christianity. This is especially true in regard to its intimate relationship with the Eastern Roman Empire from the fourth century to the demise of the empire in the fifteenth century. Also known as Byzantium, the Eastern Roman Empire affirmed Eastern Christianity as its primary spiritual inheritance. For over a millennium Orthodox Christianity was the soul of a magnificent, multifaceted Byzantine civilization. It

3

should not surprise us that much of what is described in this book reflects that important period in the church's life.

It should also be made clear that Orthodox Christianity provoked similarly close relationships with other cultures and heritages: in particular, the Arabic and the Slavic cultures. In addition, however, Orthodoxy has lived many of its years, and in many places, as a minority faith, oftentimes under severe persecution and oppression. Nevertheless, it has kept a vivid sense of the interrelationship of the holy with the valuable parts of the wisdom of the world. Without question, this effort at integration of the Orthodox Christian faith with concrete historical, social, economic, intellectual, and scientific traditions must be appreciated if the attitudes of Orthodox people toward issues of health and medicine are to be understood.

ROOTEDNESS IN TRADITION

A most important characteristic of Orthodox Christianity is its sense of tradition, that is, its rootedness in history and its sense of continuity with the past, especially the sacred past. Other characteristics are equally important, but this sense of the place of tradition colors them all. In many ways the tradition of faith and its embodiment in concrete events, writings, and cultural expressions has strong normative control over how Orthodox Christians face life today.

This sense of identity with the past may appear to contrast with the contemporary technological mind-set that looks primarily to the "new," toward discovery and progress. Some Orthodox believers have indeed fossilized the past and reject nearly everything the modern world presents. But this is not the way of the majority of Orthodox Christians, including the officialdom of the church. A dynamic quality in Orthodox teaching and lifestyle allows ready connections to be drawn between practices and decisive events of the past and contemporary developments. Most Orthodox people understand the past to contain within it the seeds of the future and the future to be grounded in the present and the past. However, the past also provides for the Orthodox a standing place by which it evaluates and critiques the present. There is neither a wholesale rejection of the accomplishments of the present nor an uncritical acceptance, just because it is new, of all that comes forth. This dual view has specific applicability to issues in health and medicine and dominates the pattern of the approach of the Orthodox church to the modern medical scene, as we shall see.

For this reason we need to look at the history of Eastern Orthodox Christianity in its relationship to its own roots, and in its connection with other religions and other forms of Christianity.

TWO MILLENNIA OF HISTORY

People who visit Orthodox church buildings find much that is unfamiliar. Frequently, questions are asked about its architecture—about the bishop's throne, for example. Those responding are frequently required to begin their explanation by referring to early Christian practices over a long range of history: from the Bible through the life of the church's persecution at the hand of the Roman Empire, to its triumph of acceptance and dominance in the same empire, to its spread throughout the world, to its relations with "separated brethren," to its subjugation to alien faiths and nations, to the renewal of its freedom, and to its place in the modern world. We speak of an almost two-thousand-year historical trek. What Orthodox Christians do, think, and perceive today is intimately related to that history and their present consciousness of identity with it. Their present cannot be understood apart from their past.

The Orthodox tell their story from their own point of view. Readers who identify with other traditions, in particular the Roman Catholic and Protestant traditions, may find the telling of this story at variance with their own historical understandings. But it is precisely in the telling of their own story as they see it that Orthodox Christians can help persons of other backgrounds to understand them, and vice versa.

This might be illustrated by an experience I had as a graduate student during a course in comparative theology in a liberal Protestant school of theology that was part of a large urban university. I was asked by the professor to make a forty-minute presentation on the Orthodox church. The last ten minutes of the hour were dedicated to questions from the class. During my presentation I had repeatedly referred to the "Fathers of the Church" as authorities for the Orthodox. The first questioner asked me to identify these "Fathers." I vividly remember wondering how someone could be a theological student and not know who the church fathers were, that is, the saintly teachers and writers of the church who had expressed the mind of the church in their lives and in their teachings and who had been acknowledged as spiritual authorities by the whole church. Most had lived before the eighth century.

When further challenged to identify some of these Fathers, I named several of the best-known from the fourth century: St. John Chrysostom, St. Basil the Great, and St. Gregory the Theologian. I was totally unprepared for what followed: the class burst out in laughter! Disturbed by this reaction, I struggled to understand it for several days, until finally the matter became clear to me. The students had laughed because their sense of the church was essentially limited to the here and now. Chrysostom, Basil, and Gregory were dead, and the church they belonged to was also dead. It was long gone and essentially irrelevant to their experience of the Christian faith.

But for me as an Orthodox Christian, Chrysostom, Basil, and Gregory are contemporaries; we belong to the same church, they are my teachers, my guides to the Scriptures, to doctrinal formulation, to worship, and to theological perspective and understanding. Eastern Orthodoxy is precisely "the Church of the Scriptures and the Fathers." As an Orthodox Christian, I view the biblical personages and the church fathers as alive and vividly present to my personal experience of the Christian faith, the Old Testament saints, the apostles, the martyrs, and the Christian saints of every kind throughout history. Above all, through the sacramental life and the mystical spiritual tradition of Orthodoxy, Christ is also a living contemporary. Nearly every feast in the church celebrating an event in the life of Christ is observed with hymns which begin "Today. . . . " Thus the church senses the birth of Christ, his transfiguration, his crucifixion, and his resurrection not simply as historical events located in the past, but as very present events in which the church and its members share "today."

Beginnings and Persecution. Orthodox Christianity is not able to identify any founder in history other than Jesus Christ and his apostles. It reveres many other holy persons, but it does not understand them as founders. There is no equivalent to a Martin Luther or a John Calvin, for instance, in the self-understanding of the Orthodox. During the first three centuries when Christianity was a persecuted religion, thousands of martyrs to the faith provided a foundation of blood upon which the young church grew. Such early writings as the *Teaching of the Twelve Apostles,* the letters of Clement of Rome and Ignatius of Antioch, and the *Epistle of Barnabas* gave witness to organized religious life, with clergy and laity involved in worship, teaching, and service. The church's strong sense of identity marked its contrast with the surrounding world. Early Christian writers known as the Apologists sought to defend the faith in a time of persecution, even writing to the highest political figures in defense of the right of Christians to maintain and practice their faith.

Freedom and Expansion. In 313 C.E. the co-emperors of the Roman Empire, Constantine and Licinius, issued the Edict of Milan which accorded to Christianity a legal status, thus allowing the church to promulgate its faith unhindered. Several years later, when Constantine was proclaimed the only emperor, he moved the capital from the ancient city of Rome to a Greek city on the border of Europe and Asia, Byzantium. He renamed the

city after himself and built it into a magnificent center of imperial authority which rivaled ancient Rome, but with this important difference: its soul
was no longer pagan but Christian.

Constantinople was then roughly in the geographical center of the empire with the Asian provinces to the east, the Mediterranean to the west,
the Arabic and Egyptian provinces to the south, and central and southeastern Europe to the north. Within a few years Christianity had made great
strides in gaining followers, and several cities had become major centers of
Christian activity and authority. The church functioned from the apostolic
period with a form of self-government based on councils. These developed
into a system of local, regional, and finally universal or "ecumenical" councils. But integral to them was the institution of the episcopacy: the bishops
of the church were the day-to-day liturgical agents of its unity, the conserv-
ers and teachers of the faith, and the administrators of its life.

By the fifth century five centers of Christian authority and organization
had come into being, with the bishops of the chief cities of those geographical areas acknowledged as their theological, liturgical, and administrative
heads. Known as the system of the pentarchy, they were ranked in order as
follows: Rome (the first capital of the empire), Constantinople (the "new
Rome"), Alexandria, Antioch, and Jerusalem.

The "East" and the "West." Although one of these centers, or patriarchates as they came to be known, was in the western part of the Mediterranean region, the other four were grouped in its eastern part. During the
fifth, sixth, and seventh centuries barbarian tribes coming out of Asia and
northern Europe repeatedly attacked the empire. In the East, a strong
military presence combined with a policy of settlement and tribute pay-
ments by the Byzantines was more successful in containing their disruptive
impact. But in the West, the Germanic and Asian tribes overran the empire repeatedly, eliminating effective government authority and introducing a long period of political, social, cultural, and economic instability. The
only source of unity, stability, and culture that enjoyed wide respect in the
West was the patriarchate of Rome, which later came to be called the papacy. Contact between East and West existed, but it became increasingly
infrequent. Christendom as a result was being slowly divided.

While Rome assumed ever greater authority and influence in this cha-
otic situation, it also began to understand the Christian faith more and
more within the context of Latin ideas, particularly in the context of Roman law. In the West the Roman patriarchate gradually became the pre-
eminent and universal authority in ecclesiastical as well as civil and
cultural matters. In the East, however, the older pattern of dealing with

the life of the church through the means of the council remained the norm, along with the mutual recognition of the four patriarchates of the East, even though the patriarch of Constantinople was in practice the most influential. The earlier traditions of faith and worship, as they had been formulated in a more Greek cultural context, were preserved in the East. As the years went by, contact decreased between a thriving Eastern Christendom and a struggling West that was seeking to absorb and christianize huge numbers of non-Roman converts. Two significantly different approaches to the Christian faith were in the making.

Schism. By the ninth century conflicts in jurisdiction, faith, liturgical practice, piety, and general outlook began to surface. More concretely, the East perceived developments in the Western part of the church as "innovations" that distorted the commonly received Christian faith. Thus in jurisdiction there were disputes over the papal claims to primacy and later the rise of Uniatism (Eastern-rite Catholicism) with its own distinctive practices;[2] in the doctrine of the Trinity, the introduction of the teaching that the Holy Spirit proceeds from the Son as well as from the Father (that is, the *filioque* doctrine); in liturgical practice, the use of unleavened bread in the Eucharist and the limitation of the sacrament of unction to the dying; in piety, enforced clergy celibacy, differing fasting practices, and the introduction of indulgences and new mariological doctrines (the Immaculate Conception); and generally a more legalistic, authority-focused understanding of the Christian life.

On several occasions conflicts led to temporary formal divisions. In the ninth century Patriarch Photius of Constantinople and Pope Nicholas I of Rome engaged in mutual excommunications, and in the first decade of the eleventh century Patriarch Sergius of Constantinople decided not to commemorate the pope in formal prayer (that is, in the diptychs—the lists kept by each hierarch of the bishops with whom he considers himself to be in communion). In 1054 a particularly sharp break occurred when papal representatives left a document of excommunication on the altar table of the Cathedral of the Holy Wisdom in Constantinople. The split, or schism, of the church into Eastern and Western entities was made final (emotionally, spiritually, and formally) in 1204, when Crusaders conquered Constantinople and for a period of time sought to suppress the Eastern Christian form of the faith and to substitute for it Latin Christianity. A half century later, the Latins were expelled, and the division was made permanent. It was then that we began to speak of two churches, the Roman Catholic church and the Eastern or Greek Orthodox church.

Western Christianity—Roman Catholicism and Protestantism. The papacy's growing power provoked both political and religious reaction. Nation-states sought to curb the temporal authority and influence of the papal church, while other groups sought to reform perceived abuses and errors. In the sixteenth century these movements came to a head in the efforts of Martin Luther in Germany and John Calvin in Switzerland, causing a division within Western Christendom: the Reformation and the rise of Protestantism. From the Orthodox perspective, then, both Roman Catholicism and Protestantism are institutions and phenomena of Western Christianity.

Threats to Eastern Orthodoxy. In the East, another course of events brought about an even sharper division between Eastern and Western Christianity: the rise of Islam. On the one hand, Eastern Christianity grew, through its missions to the Slavic peoples of the Balkans, the Ukraine, and Russia. Millions of believers were added to Orthodoxy, and a vigorous melding of Orthodox faith and Slavic cultural traditions provided a new and invigorating expression of Eastern Christianity in southeastern Europe and Asia. But concurrently the relentless drive of Islam under Arab and Turkish leadership from the seventh to the fifteenth centuries gradually forced huge Orthodox Christian populations to live under the alien control of another religion. With the fall of Constantinople to the Turks in 1453, Orthodox Byzantium's thousand-year history came to an end.

New Oppressions. For approximately four centuries, Orthodox Christians lived as second-class citizens, struggling to survive in what became known as the Muslim Ottoman Empire. The costs were very great, exemplified not only in the lives of the neomartyrs but in a widespread lack of education, economic oppression, and the development of a ghetto mentality among the enslaved peoples of Greek, Arab, Albanian, Bulgarian, Romanian, Serbian, and Slovak backgrounds. Yet they managed to survive as a faith and as peoples. In Russia, the only free Orthodox land during this period, another kind of oppression took place: Tsar Peter the Great assumed power in Russia in 1689 and spent the next thirty-six years adapting his nation and the Russian Orthodox church to Western ways of thinking and practice. The patriarchate was abolished, and until the Revolution of 1917 when the Bolsheviks took over, a concerted effort to westernize the Russian church was state policy.

The Effects of Ethnic Division and Atheistic Socialism. With the slow dissolution of the Muslim Ottoman Empire in the early 1800s, new nations appeared: Greece, Albania, Bulgaria, Romania, Serbia (Yugoslavia), and

Czechoslovakia. In each of these the Orthodox were then organized into local ethnic churches. So, for example, the Orthodox in the new state of Greece were administratively separated from the patriarchate of Constantinople and given self-governing (autocephalous) status.

Following the Russian Revolution in 1917 and the assumption of power by the Soviets, the whole of the Orthodox church in the Soviet Union suffered severe limitations on its freedom to function and has repeatedly been subject to persecution and antireligious propaganda. Nevertheless, it still survives as the largest of the Orthodox churches, with perhaps 90 million adherents.

Similar descriptions exist for the Orthodox in other Balkan nations, in the Near East, and in several African nations. Today, Orthodoxy lives and survives in nearly all of the "mother countries" in a variety of conditions, many of them repressive in different degrees. Perhaps only the Orthodox Church of Greece and the Orthodox Church of Finland enjoy a measure of freedom that Americans would consider normal.

Orthodoxy in the Modern World. Three striking phenomena characterize Eastern Orthodoxy during the twentieth century. The first is the remarkable spread of Orthodoxy through emigration from the "mother countries" to Western European countries like Germany, France, and England and to Scandinavia. But even more remarkable is the emigration to nearly all of the world's continents, most notably to North and South America. This "Orthodox diaspora" has made Orthodoxy a worldwide religion.[3]

A second phenomenon has been the freeing of Orthodox thinking and spirituality from Western influence and categories of thought (introduced into Orthodoxy primarily by Tsar Peter the Great through his so-called reforms) and a return to authentic sources of Orthodox worship, spirituality, and doctrine. Marked by the motto "Return to the Fathers!" new vigor and zeal has expressed itself in a refreshed mission activity, a developing social concern, an inspired liturgical life, and a new focus on spirituality. Paradoxically, this new direction came to be accepted precisely as Orthodox Christians moved into the "Western" world. In fact, it might be said that the diaspora experience actually provoked this "return to the Fathers" and to authentic Orthodox tradition. Remaining for resolution, however, are the jurisdictional problems among the various ethnic traditions, especially in the traditionally non-Orthodox lands.

The third phenomenon of Orthodoxy in the modern world has been its ecumenical outlook. The Orthodox have recently reaffirmed their commitment to working for Christian unity and for the improvement of relations with other religions and with those not committed to any religious tradition. With participation—within the limits imposed by doctrinal, canonical, and liturgical requirements—in the World Council of Churches, regional and national and local councils of churches, and other forms of ecumenical cooperation, Orthodox Christianity witnesses in a new way in the world at large. For the Orthodox, the center and heart of that witness is its faith and worship.

· 2 ·
Faith, Ethos, and Experience

The term *orthodox* in many American circles is used pejoratively, often referring to those who are conformist, authoritarian, static, prejudiced, ungracious, and conventional. In such a perception, to be orthodox means that one is not forward-looking, open, generous, accepting, or creative— all approved characteristics in contemporary American society. Eastern Orthodox Christians, however, are mystified by such judgments. For them, being an Orthodox Christian carries none of those negative connotations and certainly precludes none of the virtues mentioned above.

The word *orthodox* is formed out of two Greek words: *orthe* and *doxa*. The first means "correct," "accurate," "authentic." *Doxa* is understood as referring to both faith and worship. The Eastern church sees itself as manifesting the faith and worship of the undivided Christian church of the first eight centuries of the Christian era. Because its faith is, as we shall see below, built on a presupposition of dynamic growth and development, its people make these affirmations in a genuine spirit of humility, knowing well that only rarely do they fully express this "true faith" and "true worship." Rather, they find themselves in a pattern of never-ending growth and development toward God-likeness.

THE FAITH OF THE ORTHODOX

What does the Orthodox church believe? In what doctrinal teachings does it witness to the Christian truth as it is understood and lived in the Orthodox faith tradition? This question can be given only the most cursory answer here, but certain themes will later be developed more fully because of their immediate application to specific topics concerning the church's relationship with issues of health, sickness, healing, and medicine.[1]

Knowledge of God. Orthodox Christianity appreciates the search for knowledge by human beings, so it has always been open to philosophical inquiry, education, and, yes, even scientific study. Nevertheless, little can be learned about God and ultimate reality from these sources. We know about God because God reveals himself to us. He has not revealed himself to us, in the first instance, in ideas or in literature, but rather in persons. But most significantly, God has revealed himself to us as a community of persons: as a creating Father, as a saving Son, as a sanctifying Holy Spirit.

Witnesses to this self-disclosure of God are the holy Scriptures and the holy Tradition of the church, which are always held together as two witnesses to the same source of divine truth. Each interprets the other, and together they provide a coherent body of belief, which the church calls its doctrine or dogma, its axiomatic foundational teaching. The doctrinal teaching—embodied in the Bible, the decisions of the church in councils, the writings of the church fathers, the liturgical texts of the church, its canons and ethical prescriptions, the great monastic tradition with its discipline and spirituality, and, in general, the church's ethos and mind-set— is the heart of Eastern Orthodox Christianity. (It should be noted that as a result of this rootedness in the history of divine revelation, the Orthodox church rejects modernist theologies that use feminine names for God, an effort that reflects neither holy Scripture nor holy Tradition.)

God as Trinity and One. God has let us know that he is a community of persons, a holy and divine Trinity. At the same time, he has revealed that he is one reality (one God, not three). Consequently, what we know about God transcends our normal categories of knowledge which we base on our experience of the material world. What we know about God is therefore a paradox. As holy Trinity, God—the ultimate reality above and beyond the world that we experience—is personal, is in fact a community of persons. As One, God is all-knowing, all-wise, all-powerful, eternal, everywhere present, just, compassionate, and loving—the source of all that is good.

Creator and Creation. Eastern Orthodox theology both distinguishes and relates the Creator with the creation. As Creator, God is sharply distinguished in his very being from all that he has created. To be created means to be essentially and fundamentally different from the Creator: no essential analogy exists between God and what he has created. The creation functions in large part on the basis of its inner, God-given structure and inherent rules, which are maintained in effectiveness by God's continuous "energies" or grace. Thus although the creation can be studied objectively, it is only within the larger context of divine creativity that it exists and functions. This allows for scientific study of the world and concurrently for openness to God's activity in the created world. This, too, is a paradox and a mystery of faith.

The Human Condition. The Orthodox church makes a positive assessment of human potentiality. On the one hand, the church understands the creation of humanity "in the image and likeness of God" as an affirmation of all that distinguishes human beings from the rest of the created world. On the other hand, this same creation is seen as having the potential for the fulfillment of human life and capabilities by way of communion with God, so that as much as it is possible for humans, we may become God-like.

The focus of the doctrine of "original sin" is on the distortedness of the human condition as we experience it in our empirical existence, rather than on guilt. Our human condition is seen as the direct result of the break of communion between God and his creation. Separated from God, we experience our condition as a distortion of the "image" and the loss of the potential for human fulfillment, that is, the "likeness." This condition of sin in human life is characterized as "death" and "darkness." The fallen condition in which we find ourselves is the fount of human "inhumanity," sin, suffering, and misery, both personal and social.

A Savior and Salvation. The central affirmation of the Orthodox church is that out of love for humanity, God the Father sent his Son, the second person of the Trinity, into the world to take on human nature for the salvation of humanity. In the Incarnation, Jesus Christ unites the divine and the human in his one person, bridging the division. Through his teaching, his moral and spiritual guidance, and especially his death on the cross and his resurrection from the dead, Jesus Christ saved us. That is, he conquered, in principle, the power of "death" (sin, evil, distortion, imperfection, and division) in human life. Christ is thus the Savior of humanity, the victor over death. He is the light of life, dispelling spiritual darkness. Each human life is brought into communion with divine life by the Holy Spirit, the third person of the Trinity. For this reason it is called by the church the "life-giving Spirit."

The "Place" of Salvation. The church is where all this is made real for people. Through personal faith and participation in the life of the church, each person appropriates for himself or herself what Christ has done for all humanity. The church incorporates the believer into the life of the kingdom of God. It reestablishes and maintains the essential communion of each person with God in whose image we are created. Yet it does not do so automatically or magically. Each person must make continuing self-determining choices to grow toward God-likeness and to manifest ways of behavior appropriate to the kingdom of God. The Christian does this personally and corporately. Life in the church is precisely this process of growth toward God-likeness.

Worship, Spirituality, and Moral Life. "Life in the church" begins with the sacramental life. Sharing in it personalizes the salvation accomplished in Jesus Christ, makes it one's own. Baptism initiates it, causing our fallen nature to die and "resurrecting" the baptized person into a "new creation," forgiven and open to growth in God's image. The sacrament of the Eucharist continuously manifests the communion of the faithful with God and makes God's kingdom personally real. The other sacraments draw various aspects of life into the life of the kingdom. For example, matrimony incorporates marriage into kingdom living; unction draws sickness and suffering into communion with God for healing.

Orthodox spirituality is not mere piety but the discipline and means by which growth in the life of faith toward the potential fulfillment of the divinelike image in us is accomplished. With God's grace leading, followed by our repentance, prayer, and worship, our struggle against evil, the exercises for virtue—especially love—and disciplines like fasting, the salvation given us in Christ is realized and implemented. As such, morality is an integral part of spirituality and an essential element in becoming truly human, that is, God-like. All this takes place within the corporate context of the church and "in the world."

The Last Things. At some unknown point in the future, the world as we know it will be ended by God; Christ will return to judge the world and inaugurate the fullness of his kingdom. We know almost nothing of the details of this forthcoming event. We do know that our task is to be perpetually spiritually ready to meet our Maker. The church honors those who have successfully done this already—its saints—in icons, prayers, and worship services. And it continually seeks their intercessions before the throne of God. It also prays for all others who have passed on and who await the consummation of the kingdom with us. The Orthodox church thus looks upon death as an enemy which has been "conquered" in principle by Christ and which will in the future be fully overcome. It therefore addresses death and dying in a spirit of hope.

THE ORTHODOX ETHOS

Several qualities emphasized in the Orthodox faith form a pattern that sets this tradition apart from others. To capture these in words would require a combination of intellectual precision, historical grasp, spiritual wisdom, perceptive insight, and poetic talent rarely met in one person. My own attempt therefore is not exhaustive or definitive, but it should provide a measure of insight for understanding the Orthodox ethos.

The Sense of the Holy. Nothing, perhaps, characterizes Orthodox Christianity more fully and completely than its worship, which embraces at once both the transcendent and the immanent. The former conveys the sense of a reality that is beyond and above our mundane experience: the holy versus the sinful, the perfected as opposed to the fallen and distorted, the eternal as contrasted to the temporal. On the other hand, immanence gives the sense of God's closeness to the created world and all within it, of the sacred potential of ordinary life, the awareness that common and ordinary things may be vehicles of the sacred.

In Orthodox worship the first impression many people receive is that only transcendent otherworldliness is being conveyed. Unquestionably, this dimension is being emphasized. The worshipper perceives that all of life—everything genuinely important to human existence—is from God and finds its fulfillment and completion in God. Thus Orthodox worship seeks to manifest on earth a vision of the eternal kingdom of God. It is a window into heaven.

The Incarnational Sense. But together with the transcendent sense is also a sense of immanence, which readily perceives that the spiritual may be incarnated in the material, that created reality is an appropriate carrier of the holy, that matter is essentially good. Central to this affirmation is the doctrine of the Incarnation of Jesus Christ. In Christ, the divine nature remains completely and fully divine; the human, a created nature, remains always a creature. The divine is not changed to a creature; the human does not lose its humanness. But in Orthodox doctrine the divine and the human in Jesus Christ form only one person; the doctrine of the Incarnation speaks of a close coexistence of the spiritual and the material.

This pattern is extended to worship practices and beyond them into ordinary life. For example, the icon, a religious painting on a wood panel, points beyond itself to the spiritual realities it represents. It thus combines in itself both spiritual truth and this-worldly material reality. Each sacrament unites, but does not confuse, the spiritual and the material, manifesting in its special forms (water, bread, wine, oil, movements, and so on) the life of the kingdom of God.

The Transfigurational Sense. Rather than producing a static outlook, the Orthodox emphasis on both transcendent and immanent realities, coupled with the incarnational vision, gives a sense of the direction in which things should move. The transcendent should come to dwell in the common and ordinary aspects of life. Thus the human body is properly the temple of the Holy Spirit; human endeavors are to find their purpose in transcendent goals, which need to be realized, however, in the present, in the here and now. This means that the "human condition" must be in a process of change, so as to be transfigured and reformed to reflect true human purpose. Built into the Orthodox ethos, therefore, is an ongoing vision of change and development, of growth toward "God-likeness." While for Orthodoxy tradition is central, the tradition itself does not convey only a loyalty to the past but also a dynamic openness to human potential. In Orthodoxy there is a concurrent paradoxical emphasis on permanence and change.

The Sense of Evil and Sin. There is nothing Pollyannaish, however, about this sense of growth and progress toward human fulfillment. The sense of evil and sin is powerfully present in the Orthodox worldview. The sense of the distortedness of humanity's fallen condition extends to the material creation as well. None of our social institutions, nor our physical environment, nor even our minds and bodies are free from the demonic and the sinful. As we shall see below, th⟨i⟩s realistic assessment influences the Orthodox church's views on issues in health and medicine and guides its approach to the moral questions that touch on life and death. There is moral and spiritual optimism in Orthodoxy, but it is not blind or facile.

The Sense of Ultimate Victory. "Jesus Christ is victorious" could well be the motto of Orthodox Christianity. Jesus is at the center of the tradition's two major feasts: Christmas celebrates his incarnation, and Easter exalts his resurrection. The Orthodox understanding of the crucifixion of Christ is inseparable from its focus on the resurrection. The death of Christ on the cross is apprehended as an apparent victory for death, evil, sin, Satan. The resurrection is interpreted as Christ's victory over these same enemies of humanity and the creation. Without Easter, there is no salvation.

The centrality of the resurrection faith for the Orthodox is vividly clear in their midnight paschal service. Shortly before midnight, all the lights in the church are extinguished, symbolizing the darkness of the world under the sway of evil and sin. Precisely at midnight, the priest comes forth from the altar area with a lighted candle, inviting all in attendance to receive the light of the resurrection. Soon the whole church is ablaze with candlelight as each parishioner holds a lighted taper. In the "light of the Resurrection" which "fills the world," the priest goes to the center of the church and reads a Gospel passage describing the angel's triumphant announcement of the resurrection, "Why do you seek the living among the dead? He is not here. He is risen!" The whole congregation then joins in singing the hymn of the day: "Christ is risen from the dead, by his death, Death destroying; and to those in the tombs, He gives life." If any one hymn captures the spirit of the Orthodox ethos, it is this one. The Orthodox then exchange a joyous greeting for the next forty days: "Christ is risen!"— "Truly he is risen!" For the Orthodox faith, the most important thing that can be said about human existence is that "Jesus Christ is victorious!"

The Sense of Compassion and Love. Though Orthodox Christianity has clear doctrinal positions and a documented history of ethical teaching, its spirit is not dominated by rules and rigid sanctions. Rather, the compassion of God, the love of Christ, and the spirit of philanthropy dominate. This, too, is a paradox. Standards and norms, when stated alone by the Orthodox, are strict and demanding. However, when these are incorporated by the Orthodox into the perspective that all persons are called to grow in God's image, that "God is love" by biblical definition, that continuous repentance is an essential aspect of Orthodox spirituality, and that the primary virtue is love (understood as philanthropy), there is no legalism to its ethos. Compassion rules.

EXPERIENCING ORTHODOXY

When asked to describe their understanding and experience of the Orthodox faith, most Orthodox Christians are not fully articulate about doctrines and beliefs. Though the doctrines and the ethos described above form the bedrock of Orthodox experience, most laity live their Orthodox faith in more concrete ways: through their worship, sacramental life, home life, spirituality, and national heritage. But an element of tension is also part of their experience—a tension between their faith commitment and the larger society.

Since most Orthodox Christians in the U.S. are either immigrants or descendants of immigrants, the concrete embodiment of the Orthodox faith is ethnically determined in large part. These Orthodox communities—Greek, Russian, Arabic, Romanian, and so on—experience tensions between their traditions and those of the dominant culture. Even the predominant Christianity which they encounter is Western in tradition. For example, in most years the celebration of Christ's resurrection falls on a different date in the Eastern and Western traditions. Orthodoxy is a minority faith tradition distinct in many ways from the formative American religious traditions. The Orthodox person living in the U.S. thus senses a heightened contrast with the surrounding culture and also a pressure to conform with the practices of the larger society.

Orthodoxy is a church of *worship*, a highly liturgical worship. Experiencing the Divine Liturgy (the Eucharist, or the service of Holy Communion) each Sunday in the same way conveys to the worshipper a strong sense of transcendence and holiness. But worship is also associated with the changing calendar. In village life, important agricultural events like planting and harvesting were often timed to coincide with feast days of the church. For example, in Greece the beginning of the grape harvest is related to the Feast of the Transfiguration of Our Lord, August 6. Even the clergy of the church are understood by the people primarily in liturgical terms. The clergyman is not primarily an authority figure, nor a counselor, nor even an enforcer of morality. Rather, he exists essentially for the liturgical life of the church.[2]

The services convey meaning through the senses, so as to manifest symbolically the life of the kingdom of God on earth. During Holy Week, for example, the faithful relive through dramatic liturgical rites the betrayal, trial, crucifixion, death, burial, and resurrection of Christ.

Throughout the church building are visible objects that convey the spirit of holiness. An icon screen, or iconostasis, separates the altar area from the sanctuary. Icons may be found on the walls and ceiling. As one enters the church, icons are reverenced and candles lighted. The smell and sight of incense offered during the services are a call to prayer. Richly colored vestments are worn by the clergy and processions made. Special services ending with the distribution of flowers or bread or boiled wheat occur frequently. Chanting and music in modes different from the ordinary join in Orthodox worship to manifest the life of the kingdom of God on earth. Thus the transcendence of God and God's ready presence in common life are affirmed together in many ways in the worship life of the Orthodox church.

The life of an Orthodox believer is punctuated by *sacramental experience*. Brought into the community of faith by baptism in infancy, Holy Communion is administered immediately, so that an Orthodox Christian can never remember a time when he or she was not a communicating member of the church. As one grows, other services, in addition to the weekly Divine Liturgy, are important, such as the popular healing sacrament of holy unction, the memorial services for the deceased held on the forty-day, six-month, and yearly anniversaries, and the remembrance of all the dead at fixed times during the year, such as just before Pentecost. On feast days, bread-blessing services thank God for material and spiritual blessings. An impressive Service of Crowning celebrates marriage and the beginning of a new Christian family in the community. Forty days after the birth of a child, and before baptism, the mother and the child are "churched" in a rite reminiscent of the Presentation of Christ at the temple. Everyone has a "saint's day" which is noted by community and family.

Many religious practices take place *in the home*. In each proper Orthodox Christian home stands a worship center with a vigil light and icons of Christ, the Theotokos (Virgin Mary), and the patron saints of family members. The mother may cense the house daily or weekly. During lenten periods, and before Holy Communion, fasting takes place (the household abstains from foods like meat, fish, and dairy products). Many families pray at meals as well as at other times. Special baking and cooking traditions are connected with church feasts. For example, among some Orthodox a certain sweet bread is baked at New Year; only one member of the family will get the coin hidden in it, with its promise of good luck throughout the year. For some Orthodox, lamb is the preferred meal at Easter. Red dyed eggs are cracked by all in attendance around the paschal dinner table, and joyous is the one whose egg remains intact. The egg is symbolic of the resurrection—Christ "breaks out" of the tomb, as a chick breaks out of the egg. The red emphasizes Christ's joyous and "royal" victory over death, sin, and evil.

Many of these traditions are incorporated into national heritages.[3] Few Orthodox are able to separate their religious faith from their ethnic identity. Most of the European Orthodox feel that they owe their national independence to the unifying power of the Orthodox church during the period of the Muslim Ottoman domination. It was the church that kept alive national languages, traditions, and popular culture. Though inaccurate, many a Greek in earlier times would say that to be Greek was to be Orthodox and to be Orthodox was to be Greek, a phenomenon observed among other Orthodox peoples as well. It is hard to tell, in many cases, where the religious identity ends and the ethnic identity begins.

This, of course, has caused identity problems for most Orthodox in the diaspora, and in particular in America, given the dominant presence of Western Christianity.[4] Because the Orthodox are neither Roman Catholics nor Protestants, they are left out of so-called inclusive statements referring to "all Americans" as "Protestants, Catholics, and Jews." Their long history of association with ethnic traditions also tends to marginalize them.

At the same time, their inherent "incarnational ethos" moves them toward integration into the American milieu, toward the "Americanization of Orthodoxy." Social dynamics like mixed marriages accelerate the process and make demands for acculturation all the more insistent. Both laity and leadership sense tensions mounting, while most Orthodox ethnic jurisdictions adopt to a greater or lesser degree such moderating policies as bilingualism in worship, that is, the use of English in worship with Greek,

Slavonic, Arabic, Romanian, Bulgarian, and so on, continued as a liturgical language, according to each tradition.

Even more profound is the question whether it is possible to relate the Orthodox ethos to the dynamics of the American individualistic, technological, and increasingly materialistic life-style. The Orthodox are reaching out to American society in prophetic judgment and evaluation of these trends.[5] Paradoxically, the greatest promise for the perpetuation of Orthodox Christianity in America rests in the American traditions of freedom and acceptance of pluralism. These traditions are essential for the future of Orthodoxy, as a minority religion in America.

Orthodoxy, however, cannot be understood as a monolithic or inflexible life-style. Specific Orthodox people incorporate into their lives the Orthodox faith, style, and ethos, the "sense" of life and truth, in various concrete ways. No one does so absolutely; some, who are only nominally Orthodox, seem oblivious.

Nevertheless, health care professionals will find in all of their Orthodox patients something of the Orthodox Christian "sense"—a sense of life and its holiness, of sacramental appreciation for the confluence of spirit and matter and of body and soul. The evil and distortedness of sickness are acknowledged, but as long as faith is maintained, an underlying personal sense of overcoming will prevail. Religion will be experienced liturgically, in family life, in a sense of belonging to a people, a culture, and a nation. Orthodox people nearly always have a sense of rootedness, with a clear sense of identity.

And there will be a sense that the church has a place in the healing process; that God as healer and the physician as healer are not opposed to each other but together seek the well-being of the patient. The priest, as a representative of the worshipping community, is welcome at the bedside of the sick, offering prayer and sacrament for healing. In the balance of this book, we will look at the concern for healing shown in the history, faith, and way of life of the people who identify themselves as Orthodox Christians.

Part II

WELL-BEING AND ILLNESS

·3·

A Wholistic Perspective

The understanding of salvation in the Orthodox tradition is at the heart of its concern with health and well-being. As an experience and as a teaching in the life of the church, salvation addresses the whole of reality, the whole of the person, and the whole of religious life.

The tradition of the church—in the Bible, in its worship, and in the patristic tradition—has many ways of speaking about salvation.[1] Christ is preached and proclaimed in the different Christian churches as "the savior of the world,"[2] but the Christian world differs in understanding how Christ is Savior. In the history of the church many interpretations have appeared, nearly all based on one or another aspect of the tradition of faith and on specific scriptural emphases regarding salvation. These views are often referred to as theories of atonement.

In Eastern Orthodoxy darkness, death, sin, evil, the devil—that is, everything demonic—is contrasted with light, life, resurrection, and victory over death. The dominant understanding of salvation, reflecting the Gospel of John in the New Testament, is Christ's conquering of everything evil in the world, causing "death to die," as one Orthodox hymn puts it.

Theologian Gustaf Aulén, in his historical study of the three main types of the idea of the atonement, describes this Orthodox understanding as the "classic type," which he concludes is the authentic Christian understanding. He called his book *Christus Victor,* that is, Christ the Victor.[3] In his treatment of the classic view he quotes Irenaeus (130–200 c.e.), bishop of Lyons, who presents an early Christian understanding of salvation: "Mankind, that had fallen into captivity, is now by God's mercy delivered out of the power of them that held them in bondage. God had mercy upon His creation and bestowed upon them a new salvation through His Word, that is, Christ, so that men might learn by experience that they cannot attain to incorruption of themselves, but by God's grace only."[4] Inherent in this perspective on salvation is what Aulén calls a "realistic" view which accepts as real both the "dark, hostile forces of evil, and [God's] victory over them by the Divine self-sacrifice."[5]

25

The focus of the Orthodox church on victory over death (as the summation of all evils), though a central interpretation, does not exhaust the various dimensions of salvation, all of which are biblically rooted. These dimensions may be explored in the celebration of the Feast of the Elevation of the Holy Cross (September 14). The service of the day is filled with hundreds of allusions and references to other perceptions and understandings of salvation, composing a veritable tapestry. Here is neither homogenizing of theories nor an undue subordinating of approaches to salvation nor an unbiblical contrasting of perceptions about salvation. Rather, one after another, like icons on an iconostasis, each vision and understanding of salvation presents its own witness, providing us with a comprehensive mosaic of interilluminating understandings of salvation.

One vesper hymn sung at this feast-day service summarizes these understandings, presenting salvation successively as justification, as the deception of the devil, as release of human beings from subjugation to demonic forces, as the washing away of sin by the blood of Christ, as substitutionary redemption, as the assumption of humanity's guilt by the innocent One, as the overcoming of original sin, as the restoration of Eden, as suffering for the remission of sins, as divine condescension and mercy for the salvation of all humanity:

> Come, all you peoples, and let us venerate the blessed Wood, through which eternal justice has been brought to pass. For he who by a tree deceived our forefather Adam, is by the Cross himself deceived; and he who by tyranny gained possession of the creature endowed by God with royal dignity, is overthrown in headlong fall. By the blood of God the poison of the serpent is washed away; and the curse of a just condemnation is loosed by the unjust punishment inflicted on the Just. For it was fitting that wood should be healed by wood, and that through the Passion of One who knew not passion should be remitted all the sufferings of him who was condemned because of wood. But glory be to You, O Christ our King, for Your dread dispensation towards us, by which You have saved us all, for You are good and You love humankind.[6]

Thus we see that the approach to salvation in the Orthodox church is of a piece with all its life: it is comprehensive and inclusive and consequently avoids reducing things to a single idea or teaching. Nevertheless, a central theme of the Orthodox understanding of salvation gives it perspective and coherence. An analogy from art may be helpful. We do not have a pile of colored stone cubes, the tesserae that artists use to create a mosaic. Rather, we have a beautiful mosaic icon with pattern and form and a theme—the triumph of Christ over the forces of death and darkness—which holds all the pieces together in a unified and meaningful image.

This wholistic approach to salvation in Orthodox Christianity allows the vision of the church to encompass much more than "strictly religious" concerns. Everything in the creation is the subject of God's saving work, including the material world, and in particular, human beings in the totality of their existence.

SALVATION AS THERAPY

Salvation is not only *from* something; it is *for* something as well. The saving work of Jesus Christ has done more than conquer the devil, death, corruption, sin, and evil, the enemies of authentic human life. His saving work has promised to all in this new life a victory, whose fruits are communion with God, the source of life; communion with our fellow creatures both human and subhuman; fullness of humanity; light, goodness, truth— in short, well-being of body and soul. This renewed fullness of life is succinctly described as *theosis*, or God-likeness.

Theosis is the Orthodox name for the goal toward which human beings are called by God to move and develop. It is the fulfillment of the potential of our creation in "the image and likeness" of God. According to the Greek fathers of the church, our ability to become like God was lost through original sin, and the "image" was distorted, weakened, and darkened, but not destroyed. The potential for God-likeness was restored to us by the saving work of Jesus Christ, and movement toward its fulfillment is made possible by communion with the Holy Spirit. Growth in God-likeness occurs as human life manifests, in numerous ways appropriate to our created condition, the glory of God. Thus we grow toward theosis, "from glory to glory" (2 Corinthians 3:18) in a never fully completed process of being "transformed by the renewal of [our] mind, that [we] may prove what is the good and acceptable and perfect will of God" (Romans 12:2). Since Jesus Christ is the "firstborn among many brethren," theosis means that we are destined "to be conformed to the image of [God's] Son" (Romans 8:29), in order to become more fully human.

Because salvation leads humanity in this direction, the Eastern Christian perspective does not focus on a legal interpretation. In the description of Greek theologian Nikos A. Matsoukas, the words that best characterize the Orthodox approach to the reality of salvation are *healing* and *therapy*.

> Created life has the need to participate in that which is "life-itself" (God). This is the key position in Orthodox theology for understanding and interpreting original sin, salvation, and immortality. For this reason, given the failure of humanity to participate in the being and the well-

being of divine life, the church offers healing, since in its custody are
the goods of the work of redemption. With this medicinal terminology,
we understand the major emphases of theology. . . . [7]

In Matsoukas's interpretation, salvation is thus the "correction and therapy
of the nature of the human being, so that the human being may become a
god by grace, to participate in the divine glory."[8] At the core of Christianity
in the Orthodox church, then, is a therapeutic, healing approach.

This healing vision of God at work in the world applies primarily to the
religious, the spiritual, and the moral dimensions of life, but not exclusively
so. It forms a matrix of concern that includes every part of life,
restoring and healing the life being transfigured into one fully in communion
with God and his creation. It thus comes naturally to pray to God, "the
Physician of our souls and bodies." God, the creator of both soul and body,
is understood as the source of all healing.

Pastoral practice is strongly therapeutic. Among the Greek Orthodox,
the chanting of the Smaller Supplicatory Canon is often requested of the
priest in cases of sickness and illness. Visits to the hospital and prayers for
the sick are expected of pastors. Healing shrines continue to be integral
parts of the Orthodox tradition. These and many other practices described
in subsequent chapters are deeply rooted in the consciousness of the faithful,
both clergy and lay.

But the Orthodox church does not limit its ideas about healing the sick
to narrowly spiritual and religious spheres of activity. The healing of sickness,
as we shall see, is encouraged by this "therapeutic" faith in many
ways, not the least of which is rational medicine.

THE RELATIONSHIP OF BODY AND SOUL

One touchstone that helps define a faith tradition's relationship to issues
of health, illness, and medicine is its perceptions about the body. Although
some forms of Christianity commonly contrast body and soul sharply, Eastern
Orthodox Christianity, while not confusing them or identifying them,
sees them as united and intimately related. A letter written by St. Basil in
the fourth century to a physician friend illustrates:

Humanity is the regular business of all you who practice as physicians.
And, in my opinion, to put your science at the head and front of life's
pursuits is to decide reasonably and rightly. This at all events seems to
be the case if man's most precious possession, life, is painful and not
worth living, unless it be lived in health, and if for health we are dependent
upon your skill. In your own case medicine is seen, as it were, with

two right hands; you enlarge the accepted limits of philanthropy by not confining the application of your skills to men's bodies, but by attending also to the cure of the diseases of their souls. It is not only in accordance with popular report that I thus write. I am moved by the personal experience which I have had on many occasions.[9]

For St. Basil physical and emotional disturbances were equally within the purview of the physician. In the same manner, body and spirit are equally of concern for the Christian church. In pursuing their common goal to cure the whole person, the church will certainly use methods and means different from those of the physician. But also different is the grounding for this common concern. For the church's perspective on well-being and illness is grounded in its perception of the closeness of body and soul as integral aspects of what it means to be a human being as created by God.

A quite early Christian document presents clearly, directly, and simply the views of the church on the body itself. Around the year 347, Cyril, bishop of the church of Jerusalem, gave instruction to a group of candidates for baptism. At that time persons who wished to become Christians learned about the Christian faith in a thorough course of study during Lent and Eastertide. They were baptized on Holy Saturday and participated in the Easter liturgy. We have twenty-four of these lectures, known as the *Catecheses*, which present the faith and practice of this early Jerusalem church.

A theme treated in them is the place of the body in Christian thought. Because the audience for these lectures was not a theologically trained one, but people learning the first elements of the faith, we have here an attempt to explain what is essential in the teaching of the church. The positions stated in these lectures form the outline for examining the "mainline" Eastern Orthodox tradition regarding the body.

The Goodness of the Body. In Lecture 4, which carries the significant title "On the Dogmas," St. Cyril devotes a section to the body itself and several other sections to related topics like food, clothing, and the resurrection of the body.[10] Cyril begins his teaching by warning his audience about those who would condemn the body, who see it opposed in some ultimate sense to God and things holy: "Do not bear with anyone if he says that the body is alien to God." Cyril is thinking of false teachers who appeared early in Christian history. Holding a dualistic view of reality, they sharply contrasted its spiritual dimensions (good) with its material dimensions (evil).[11] These views had appeared in the Christian community even before the New Testament canon was complete and had been condemned already in it.[12]

In contrast, St. Cyril proceeds to lift up the body as something marvelous and rich in dignity. He presents its biological functioning as a wondrous creation of God, inspiring awe and respect.

> But why have they depreciated this marvelous body? Wherein does it fall short in dignity? What is there about its construction that is not a work of art? Ought not the alienators of the body from God to have taken knowledge of the brilliant ordaining of eyes? or how the ears are placed right and left, and so receive hearing with nothing in the way? Or how the sense of smell can distinguish one vapour from another, and receives exhalations? Or how the tongue has a double ministry in maintaining the faculty of taste and the activity of speech? How the lungs, hidden away out of sight, keep up the breathing of air with never a pause? Who established the ceaseless beating of the heart? Who distributed blood into so many veins and arteries? Who was so wise as to knot bones to muscles? Who was it that assigned us part of our food for sustenance, and separated off part to form a decent secretion (perspiration is meant by this phrase), while hiding away the indecent members in the more fitting positions? Who, when man was constituted that he will die, ensured the continuance of his kind by making intercourse so ready?[13]

Cyril's teaching was frequently repeated. Thus, according to St. Gregory Palamas, writing in the fourteenth century, "There is nothing bad in the body, since the body is not evil in itself."[14]

The Body and Sin. If the body, as a creation of God, is in principle good, then those who blame the body and its needs, desires, and impulses for the sin and evil in human life are wrong. Speaking practically and directly to his catechumens, Cyril of Jerusalem uses striking illustrations that hammer home his point.

> Do not tell me that the body is the cause of sin. For were the body the cause of sin, why does no corpse sin? Put a sword in the right hand of a man who has just died, and no murder takes place. Let beauty in every guise pass before a youth just dead, and he will not be moved to fornication. Wherefore so? Because the body does not sin of itself, but it is the soul that sins, using the body.[15]

Of course, those who taught that the body was the cause of sin could point to certain passages in the New Testament for support. For example, in Romans 7:25 St. Paul says: "I of myself serve the law of God with my mind, but with my flesh I serve the law of sin." Romans 8 seems on the surface to be exactly opposite to Cyril's teaching: " . . . those who live according to the flesh set their minds on the things of the flesh, but those who live according to the Spirit set their minds on the things of the Spirit.

To set the mind on the flesh is death, but to set the mind on the Spirit is life and peace. For the mind that is set on the flesh is hostile to God; it does not submit to God's law, indeed it cannot; and those who are in the flesh cannot please God" (verses 5–8). The unwary and careless reader could easily misunderstand these lines and conclude that anything having to do with the bodily life is opposed to God and is incapable of pleasing him.

But what is being spoken of here, in both the Scriptures and the patristic teaching, is not the body. In Greek, the word *soma* is used most often to refer to the body in a positive or ethically neutral way. The word *sarx*, frequently translated "flesh," is used in two very different ways. Often it refers to the body or human life in general, carrying with it no negative connotation, but on the contrary even a positive one. Thus "the two shall be one flesh" (Matthew 19:5); "and all flesh shall see the salvation of God" (Luke 3:6); "the Word became flesh and dwelt among us" (John 1:14); "the bread which I shall give for the life of the world is my flesh" (John 6:51); "no man hates his own flesh, but nourishes and cherishes it" (Ephesians 5:29).

But many times *sarx* carries with it the meaning of distorted and sinful passions, as in Romans 7 and 8. These "desires of the flesh" have less to do with the body itself than with sin. If "fleshly desires" (1 Peter 2:11) become dominant in a person, the church fathers speak of a condition of "fleshly mentality." This understanding helps us to interpret properly the passage in Romans 8 quoted above, and others similar to it. It is not the body itself that is hostile to God but the "mind set on the flesh," a classical definition of sin. Sin is being spoken of in these passages.

The Body as the Soul's Tool. As Cyril of Jerusalem continued his discussion of the body, he moved to the topic of its appropriate use.

> The body is the soul's tool, and also serves as a garment and robe of the soul. If then the body is given over to fornication by the soul, the body is impure, but if it cohabits with a holy soul, it is a temple of the Holy Spirit. This is not my assertion. It was Paul the Apostle that said "Know ye not that your bodies are the temple of the Holy Ghost, which is in you" (1 Corinthians 6:19). Take care, therefore, of the body, as the possible temple of the Holy Spirit. Do not pollute your flesh with fornication, and soil what is your fairest robe. But should you have polluted it, cleanse it now by penitence.[16]

Cyril's treatment of sex and marriage provides an example of his attitude toward the right use of the body. He is opposed to those rigorists who condemn sex, even marriage, and give honor only to those who have committed themselves to God in sexual abstinence. Speaking to the latter, after praising them for their commitment to the angelic life of chastity, he says, "do not make the opposite mistake of guarding chastity successfully and being puffed up with disdain of those who have come down to marrying . . . and are using [wedlock] aright." Marriage is the right place for sex. "But every other kind of sex-relation must be put right away, fornication, adultery, and every form of debauchery. The body is to be kept pure for the Lord, that the Lord may look favourably upon the body."[17] A similar approach is taken to food and clothing.

Cyril notes that both sinners and the righteous will be resurrected, though they will have different kinds of bodies from each other.[18] He holds that this is a "just disposition of God in respect of both orders, for nothing that we do is done without the body." With the mouth we may blaspheme or we may pray; with the body we are chaste or we fornicate; with the hand we steal or we give charity, he says. "Therefore, since it is the body that has served to every work, the body will have its share in what comes to pass in the hereafter."[19] Thus the body is given an eternal significance.

Orthodox Christianity does not denigrate the body, which is respected as an essential and even eternal aspect of the human condition. We are not fully human without the body, and we are obliged to use it in a way that shares in the God-like life. This takes place both in this life and in the next. The body's impulses may be the occasion for misuse and abuse. This reality of sin is the source of the biblical and monastic references to the "fleshly mind" and the attractions of the "flesh." But, equally, the body can share in the "spiritual mind" and the "life in the Spirit." How we use it is the critical point.

Care for the Body. Even as Cyril has uppermost the spiritual, ethical, and moral use of the body, he counsels the need to care for the body in a respectful manner. He has already spoken of the need to feed and clothe the body appropriately. His general conclusion about the body is of interest for our concern regarding health and medicine, though only generally stated. "So brethren," he says to those about to be baptized, "let us take good care of our bodies and not misuse them as if they were no part of ourselves. Do not let us say what the heretics say, that the body is a garment, and not part of us, but let us take care of it as being our own. For we shall have to give account to the Lord for everything we have done with the body as instrument."[20]

Care for the body, of course, does not mean indulgence of the body. It means that the body and its appetites should be under the control of the spiritual dimension of life. Oftentimes, however, critics of monastic asceticism hold that the rigors of ascetic practice—limited sleep, severe fasting, sexual abstinence, hard work, solitude, vigils, long hours of prayer, restrictions on personal cleanliness, poverty—were designed not to care for the body but to weaken and destroy it. Certainly, throughout the long history of Christian asceticism, some monks functioned in this way. Some even saw illness as a test of their ascetic resolve, a trial to be endured, and did not seek healing for themselves.[21] Nevertheless, this is not a main line of Orthodox teaching regarding ascetic discipline and its relationship to the body. Rather, all ascetic disciplines as they affect the body are perceived as means to an end—the submission of life to God's purposes and the transformation of human life into the fullness of the image and likeness of God.

Evagrius Ponticus (346–399) was one of the earliest monastics to reflect on the ascetic life. He cautioned that all ascetic practices were to be engaged in "according to due measure and at the appropriate times." Margaret Miles, a patristics scholar, summarizes his teaching thus: "Any bodily discipline must be carefully designed to address the exact nature of the spiritual distraction and not applied to the body as if to control an enemy." She adds that Evagrius, together with another early ascetic writer, John Cassian (c. 360–435), were concerned "to acknowledge the usefulness of some form of bodily discipline, but having done that, to speak against any abuse of the body." She concludes that "the ascetic who understands the 'tools of the trade' will benefit both body and soul by the ascetic practices employed."[22] Thus Evagrius tells his readers, "The human body is like a coat. If you treat it carefully it will last a long time. If you neglect it, it will fall into tatters."[23]

So long as inordinate attention is not given to the body at the expense of more important things, the care for the body is a Christian virtue and responsibility. It shares in every aspect of human existence, even the most spiritual, when it is fittingly used.

In the Eastern Orthodox tradition the body is intimately related to the spiritual dimension of life. It has a permanent and continuing significance because of its creation by God and its eventual resurrection, but also in the present life because it is to share fully in the transfiguring power of the God-like life. Thus, over a millennium and a half ago, Cyril, bishop of Jerusalem, taught his new converts a series of truths about the body which have remained "core teaching" for Eastern Orthodoxy: the body is not alien to God; the body is not in itself a cause of sin; the soul uses the body for good or for evil and may thus be not only a mere tool but a temple as well; the body is a permanent and essential aspect of the whole human nature; as a result it shares in the God-likeness to which human beings are called; and consequently, one has a responsibility to care for its well-being and health.

Such a positive view of the potentials of the body, while not ignoring the ease with which the body can be sinfully misused, avoids a division of the spiritual from the physical aspects of human life. This wholeness in turn provides a supportive and hospitable environment for serious, deliberate, and compassionate concern when illness and sickness come. Because sickness is seen as an evil to be overcome, the Orthodox perspective on evil has an important bearing on the concerns of this volume.

· 4 ·

Illness

What connection do health and illness have with the experience of evil in our lives? Every religious tradition is forced in one way or another to confront that question. Perhaps the distinctive perspective of the Orthodox Christian church is its understanding of evil as a privation of good, causing humanity to live in a distorted and fallen condition. This condition includes the empirical reality of illness. The evil of sickness, however, is not considered absolute; it can even offer opportunities for spiritual growth. The question of health and illness in human existence is thus approached as a paradox; at the same time, the tradition lays down concrete responsibilities in that sphere.

THE UNDERSTANDING OF EVIL

At the source of all Christian thinking and reflection about evil and sin is the Genesis story of Adam and Eve in the Old Testament. Certainly, it has been understood throughout the centuries of the Christian tradition as a historic event, but it has been understood as well during all this period as a description of the unredeemed state of human beings. In short, the biblical story of human creation and the fall is at heart a description of the human condition.

Where the sin of Adam is perceived primarily as disobedience of a rule or law, then sin and evil will be countered with the theme of righteousness and obedience to law. This was not the way of the Christian East. The earliest Christian tradition interpreted the story differently. The sin of the "first created" (Greek, *protoplastoi*) is perceived primarily, though not exclusively, as a willful breaking of the appropriate relationship between God and his creation by the first-created parents of the human race. The result of Adam's sin was a new condition of distortedness and corruption, of which illness and ultimate physical death were only part.

In order to grasp the Eastern Christian approach to evil, we must ask an even more fundamental question. What is the source of good in our lives, or to probe even more deeply, what is good in itself? To this philosophical question the Eastern Christian tradition knows only one answer: God. Thus, in the theological tradition of the spiritual fathers, we read repeatedly statements like these:

> From St. Maximus the Confessor: "Goodness by nature belongs to God alone, from whom all things capable by nature of receiving light and goodness are enlightened and blessed with goodness by participation."[1]

> From St. Mark the Ascetic: "First of all, we know that God is the beginning, middle and end of everything good: and it is impossible for us to have faith in anything good or to carry it into effect except in Christ Jesus and the Holy Spirit."[2]

It follows quite readily that if good is to be found in communion with God, evil is the absence of communion with God. Whatever is not in communion with God is evil. And since our fallen condition is precisely "fallen" because it is not in communion with God, our human condition participates in evil in proportion to our lack of communion with God. Evil is the distortion and corruption of the created world, its transformation from its true nature to an essentially unnatural condition.

But it would be a serious mistake to interpret this view as implying that evil, sickness, and suffering are somehow illusory. Empirically, evil is real and experienced in the created world. The condition of fallenness has a terrible impact on the human condition.

In the patristic tradition, much is said about the consequences of the break of communion and relationship with God. The will is seen as being weakened, the emotions distorted, and the mind darkened. A favorite patristic word for this condition of fallenness and distorted humanity is *corruption*. The fifth-century spiritual writer St. Diadochus of Photike expressed it thus in his treatise "On Spiritual Knowledge": "As a result of Adam's fall, not only were the main lines of the character of the soul befouled, but our body also became the subject of corruption."[3] One dimension—and by no means the most important—of that corruption is sickness.

MONASTIC INSIGHTS ON THE ABSENCE OF HEALTH

Given Eastern Orthodoxy's understanding of the close and interpenetrating relationship of body and soul, a fully healthy relationship of the soul with God would in principle provide us with a fully healthy body. Our broken communion with God, however, leads us inexorably through illness to death. In the words of St. Maximus the Confessor, sin "brought the sentence of death on all nature, since through man it impels all created things towards death."[4] Thus it follows that for the patristic theological tradition, health is the norm of the living human being, and sickness is understood as the absence of health, in a direct correspondence to the understanding of evil as the absence of the good.

Nevertheless, neither physical sickness nor physical death are the most significant dimensions of life: growth in communion with God is the Christian's goal. Although sickness is never perceived to be a good in itself, it can be approached instrumentally, as a means to the Christian's goal. Spiritual advice about illness thus takes on a relative character. The means for curing illness vary, and most are acceptable, yet every case of sickness can become a means to growth in God-likeness.

This approach to illness is most clearly seen in the teaching of the monastic fathers. Although they write for those who have given up "the world" to live only for God, the main lines of their teaching apply to all. These writers posit the view that illnesses, even when we seek to cure them, may be seen as occasions for spiritual growth, as tests of our commitment and devotion to God. St. Macarius of Egypt, an otherwise unknown monastic writer who probably lived in the late fourth or early fifth century, wrote homilies that were widely read and studied in Byzantium. A paraphrase of these, attributed to the eleventh-century St. Symeon Metaphrastes, expresses this instrumentalist view of illness under the heading "The Freedom of the Intellect":

> He who wants to be an imitator of Christ, so that he too may be called a son of God, born of the Spirit, must above all bear these, be they bodily illnesses, slander and vilification from men, or attacks from unclean spirits. God in His providence allows souls to be tested by various afflictions of this kind, so that it may be revealed which of them truly loves Him."[5]

The critical word in this quotation is *allows*. It lies at the heart of the Eastern Christian understanding that belief in a good God and the experience of human suffering can coexist. God "permits" a testing, after the fashion of Job, of even the innocent. The appropriate response is one of patience and forbearance, based on love for God and trust in him.

Consequently, health and illness can be seen as gifts from God, as instruments for the fulfilling of his purposes. Health is generally thought of as good and is to be sought after. But when it comes, illness may also be an occasion for growth in the real purpose of life for a believer. Clearly, Christians are instructed to receive everything in their lives not only with patience and forbearance but with a sense that all is a gift from God to provide opportunity for the fulfillment of spiritual potential. St. Peter of Damascus elaborates on this truth:

> We ought all of us to give thanks to God for both the universal and the particular gifts of soul and body that He bestows on us. The universal gifts consist of the . . . elements [of the creation] and all that comes into being through them, as well as all the marvelous works of God mentioned in the divine Scriptures. The particular gifts consist of all that God has given to each individual. These include wealth, so that one can perform acts of charity; poverty, so that one can endure it with patience and gratitude; authority, so that one can exercise righteous judgment and establish virtue; obedience and service, so that one can more readily attain salvation of soul; health, so that one can assist those in need and undertake work worthy of God; sickness, so that one may earn the crown of patience. . . . All these things, even if they are opposed to each other, are nevertheless good when used correctly, but when misused, they are not good, but are harmful for both soul and body.

Speaking as a monastic, Peter of Damascus continues in this passage to evaluate the gifts of God: "Better than them all, however, is the patient endurance of afflictions." The reason is clear: "he who has been found worthy of this great gift should give thanks to God in that he has been all the more blessed. For he has become an imitator of Christ, of His holy apostles, and of the martyrs and saints."[6]

Nevertheless, both health and illness are also seen as temptations to do evil. In his "Gnomic Anthology," for example, the late-eleventh-century writer Elias the Presbyter creates a distinction based on the exercise of the will: "Trials and temptations subject to our volition are chiefly caused by health, wealth and reputation; and those beyond our control by sickness, material losses and slander. Some people are helped by these things, others are destroyed by them."[7] His point is clear: both health and sickness can be used by the believer to build up the God-likeness of his or her life, but those same circumstances can also be the occasions for failure in the Christian journey. In the light of the ultimate purpose of life, neither health nor sickness is itself unambiguously good or evil.

Given this instrumentalist view, the paradox is increased when, under normal circumstances and conditions, the monk is sometimes cautioned by some spiritual writers not to seek healing in illness, and by others to do so. For example, St. Diadochus of Photike, speaking of the church in the post-Constantinian period, sees illness for the monk as a necessary element of the Christian struggle, since martyrdom is no longer available to him.[8] On the other hand, frequent counsels in the *Philokalia*, the most important collection of Eastern Orthodox monastic spiritual writings, note the monk's limited ability to do his spiritual work when he becomes physically ill. Thus Evagrius the Solitary (fourth century) is compassionate and considerate. In his discussion of the duty of monks to eat only once daily, he speaks about the monk who falls ill: "there are occasions when, because of a bodily sickness, you have to eat a second and a third time or more often. Do not be sad about this; when you are ill you should modify your ascetic labors for the time being, so that you may regain the strength to take them up once more."[9] Similarly, St. John of Karpathus counsels, "If you try to keep the rules of fasting and cannot do so because of ill health, then with contrition of heart you should give thanks to Him who cares for all and judges all."[10]

Other writers within the Orthodox tradition speak of the need to maintain health by preventive care and by seeking healing, both human and divine, when illness comes. St. John Cassian (c. 360–435), for example, counsels his monks and all Christians in practical terms: "Bodily illness is not an obstacle to purity of heart, provided we give the body what its illness requires, not what gratifies our desire for pleasure. Food is to be taken in so far as it supports our life, but not to the extent of enslaving us to the impulses of desire. To eat moderately and reasonably is to keep the body in health, not to deprive it of holiness."[11]

Perhaps the strongest affirmation of the need to care for health in the *Philokalia* comes from St. Diadochus of Photike, who instructs his monastic readers—and by extension all Christians—in the use of medicine and in some of the disciplines of spiritual healing.

There is nothing to prevent us from calling a doctor when we are ill. Since Providence has implanted remedies in nature, it has been possible for human experimentation to develop the art of medicine. All the same we should not place our hope of healing in doctors, but in our true Savior and Physician, Jesus Christ. I say this to those who practice self-control in monastic communities or towns, for because of their environment [confinement in their communities] they cannot at all times maintain the active working of faith through love. Furthermore, they should not succumb to the conceit and temptation of the devil, which have led some of them publicly to boast that they have had no need of doctors for many years. If on the other hand, someone is living as a hermit in more deserted places together with two or three like-minded brethren, whatever sufferings may befall him let him draw near in faith to the only Lord who can heal "every kind of sickness and disease" (Matt. 4:23). For besides the Lord he has the desert itself to provide

sufficient consolation in his illness. In such a person faith is always ac-
tively at work, and in addition he has no scope to display the fine quality
of his patience before others, because he is protected by the desert.[12]

Finally, the Christian has a responsibility to care for those who are sick.
The neighbor's sickness is an evil that calls for compassionate care and an
effort to heal. Sometimes the monk—as a test of endurance—did not seek
his own healing. His restraint was seen as part of the discipline he was to
live. But he never counseled this course of action to others who suffered,
especially those who were not monks. Thus caring for the sick is an aspect
of prayer, of communion with God.

APPROACHING SICKNESS

The monastic views sketched in the previous section validly represent Eastern Orthodoxy's approach to illness as an evil. Separating out
the elements distinctive to the monastic calling, we should arrive at a general understanding of Orthodox Christianity's perspective on illness and
sickness.

This perspective can be briefly stated in eleven propositions.

1. *Evil is a condition.* Ultimate reality, God, is good and the source of
all good. God is the Uncreated and is the only pure good. All creation is
good only inasmuch as it participates and communes with God. Evil comes
into being with the deliberate renunciation of communion with God; it is
therefore understood in Orthodox Christianity as "the absence of the
good." The fallen condition of the created world therefore, by definition,
means that much of existence is evil. This does not mean that the creation
itself is evil. Because of its broken relationship with God, nature is in fact
"unnatural," and human beings are in fact "less than human." We are born
into this fallen, unnatural, and less than fully human condition.

2. *Sickness is an evil.* Because of the fallen condition in which humanity finds itself, everything is subject to corruption. This does not mean that
everything is totally corrupt or that there cannot be in the fallen condition
a significant proportion of the human experience which is good. Nevertheless, only the fully natural is good. Since evil is a privation of the good,
evil is by definition unnatural. An aspect of this reality is illness. Sickness,
as a result, is fundamentally seen as part of a global disharmony, disorientation, and disorder; it is perceived as a fundamental evil integral to the
fallen experience of humanity and therefore unavoidable.

3. *The goal of life as God-likeness transforms illness.* Yet evil, and illness as a particular evil, are within the parameters of the work of salvation

of Jesus Christ. The saving work of Christ in Eastern Orthodoxy is seen as victory over the enemies of true human existence. Sickness, a discontinuity with the presence and energies of God, can be transformed into an instrument for the fulfillment of human purpose, which is to realize as fully as possible the image and likeness of God in human life.

4. *Sickness is a testing.* When the Christian suffers an illness, he or she is being tested. Illness is seen not as an absolute evil but as an evil capable of redemption, if it enhances communion with God and growth in full God-like personhood. Its proper use is the issue. In the same manner, health is not an absolute good but a test. It, too, provides opportunities either for good or for evil.

5. *Sickness is a gift.* If the test of sickness is met properly, it can force us to face up to our selves, our values, our vices and virtues. It can teach us what is truly important about our lives. It can mold our character into a more God-like pattern, and as a result it can make us more fully and more completely human. Unhealed sickness or illness under therapy can be a gift that transforms human life in the direction of fulfillment.

6. *Sickness is a temptation.* There is nothing automatic, however, about the potential of sickness to help us achieve full human purpose as the image and likeness of God. If we do not accept it as a gift from God, it can also stand as a temptation to despair, to further distancing from God, to an even sharper division between our empirical selves and our true human nature. As such, sickness is dangerous, not only to our bodily condition but to our spiritual condition. Remarkably the same can be said about health: it too is a temptation that can lead human beings far from God and from their own humanity.

7. *Illness is an occasion for witness.* Propositions 4, 5, and 6 refer to the inner disposition and inner potentialities given the Christian when he or she faces illness. The bearing of illness can also serve as a witness to others. Like a new form of martyrdom, it provides a way of giving witness to others of the faith that we hold.

8. *Illness affects other responsibilities.* As a trial, as a gift, as a temptation, as an occasion for witness, sickness becomes in itself a "calling." It is valued as a potential instrument of God's will, and as such, it morally frees the sick person from responsibility for some other duties he or she normally has. These, of course, are not abandoned, but they may recede in importance as the Christian seeks to transform the evil of sickness into growth in God-likeness.

9. *Health maintenance is a responsibility.* One ought not deliberately harm one's own health. Just as early Christians were prohibited from pro-

voking the occasions for martyrdom, so no Christian should deliberately
and without proper cause put life and health to risk. Rather, because
health is a good and illness an evil, one has a basic responsibility to preserve and maintain life and health. Reckless risking of health and life,
abusing the body, ignoring the basic necessities of life—all constitute inappropriate behavior for the Christian.

10. *It is appropriate for a Christian to seek healing when sick.* Although
sickness is not an absolute evil and can in fact become the occasion for
growth toward fullness of life, Eastern Christianity does not teach passivity
in the face of illness. We have a responsibility to seek healing, using means
ranging from the purely spiritual to the purely scientific. Traditionally,
both means are used without a sense of conflict. Spiritual healing methods, including prayer and sacraments, are applied in conjunction with "rational medicine" to effect healing. For the church, the true source of the
good of healing is God. Christ is the "physician of our souls and bodies."
In this sense, the physician is also perceived as a servant of God's will and
purposes, allowing the good of health to emerge wherever possible.

11. *Christians have a responsibility for the health of others.* An essential
dimension of Christian love, itself a chief dimension of God-likeness, is
concern for the well-being of the neighbor. No one, even the most remote
desert ascetic, can grow in God-likeness without caring for another who
suffers affliction. Because everyone eventually suffers the affliction of illness, the care of the sick is an expression of fulfilling the image and likeness of God in relationship toward others. Christians thus have a
universally acknowledged responsibility to aid others in reducing the evil
of sickness in this life.

SINS AND SICKNESS

Orthodox Christians sometimes express the idea that God has visited
them with sickness as a consequence of their sinful acts. "What have I
done that God caused me to become ill?" they may ask. The Eastern
Christian perspective, however, does not allow for a general causal relationship between particular illnesses and specific sins.

Sickness as an evil is part of the fabric of our fallen existence; as a phenomenon, it pervades the world and our existence.[13] But in most cases, we
cannot speak of a direct link between a particular sin and contracting an
illness. Rather, the corruption that pervades all of our existence and expresses itself in a myriad of ways also sets the stage for illness and finally
death.

Nevertheless, as we have seen from the tenth point in the previous section, Christians have a responsibility to care for the gift of health which they may enjoy. The critical issue is one of use and abuse. An example is the improper use of food. St. Nicetas Stethatos (fourteenth century) thus observes, "From an irregular and inappropriate diet, illnesses are frequently provoked in many people."[14] St. Maximus the Confessor points to many dimensions of life in which goodness or evil is precisely determined by proper use or improper abuse. In his "Second Century on Love" he refers to things appropriate to the soul, with "spiritual knowledge and ignorance, forgetfulness and memory, love and hate, fear and courage, distress and joy" as examples. Others, he notes, are "in the body": "pleasure and pain, sensation and numbness, health and disease, life and death." Things "relating to the body" are "having children and not having children, wealth and poverty, fame and obscurity," and the like. Their goodness or evil, however, is not intrinsic. He teaches that "according to how they are used they may rightly be called good or evil." Care and attentiveness is required so as to avoid abuse in all these things. "Do not misuse your conceptual images of things," he says, "lest you are forced to make a wrong use of the things themselves."[15]

As a result, St. Maximus finds that "immoderation and thoughtless behavior" are condemned by Christian revelation.

> Scripture does not forbid anything which God has given us for our use; but it condemns immoderation and thoughtless behavior. For instance, it does not forbid us to eat, or to beget children, or to possess material things and to administer them properly. But it does forbid us to be gluttonous, to fornicate and so on.[16]

The application of this view to health is easily made. Abuse of our health can produce illness and is therefore sinful. Some sinful behavior can be the cause of some illnesses. But not all illnesses, as we have seen, can be attributed to specific sinful behavior. For example, the abuse of narcotic drugs frequently results in mental, spiritual, and physical illness; liver ailments may be caused by the abuse of alcohol; venereal diseases are frequently contracted through sexual promiscuity; overeating may provoke heart disease, and so on. Personally committed sins, in short, may directly cause some illnesses. Hence, the Christian responsibility toward our health requires us to avoid abusing the many goods of life. We have a tendency to do this as we become subject to pleasure seeking. The wrong kind of pleasure seeking thus becomes an issue of spirituality as well as concern for health.

Inexorably, we come back to the human condition, our fallenness, our need to be in communion with God. Growing in the image and likeness of God toward *theosis* thus has its ethical ramifications for physical and mental health and illness.

·5·

Suffering

When we speak of evil, our frame of reference tends to be abstract, philosophical, cosmic. We tend to intellectualize, to see evil as a problem to be addressed by correct thinking. When we turn to the experience of evil in the lives of people and attempt to deal with it experientially, the word *suffering* seems more appropriate. Those who suffer seek to understand their condition not primarily with the mind but with the heart and soul, and their struggle evokes in others a response of compassion.

The Orthodox tradition accepts the paradoxes of suffering, holding together in life and experience that which the mind sees as contrasts and even as contradictions. By considering the tradition's distinction between voluntary and involuntary suffering, along with its views on the limiting of suffering, the inevitability of suffering, suffering as trial, and the transfiguring power of suffering, we can begin to grasp the Orthodox perspective.

INVOLUNTARY AND VOLUNTARY SUFFERING

A Greek word used to designate suffering, pain, and affliction is *thlipsis*, whose root means "to crush under a heavy weight." In its liturgical life the Orthodox church frequently prays that God protect people from that crushing weight, alleviate their sufferings, and barring that, grant comfort to those who suffer. An expression of compassion, these prayers obviously consider suffering an evil to be limited and overcome, if not eliminated.

In a paradoxical way, however, the Orthodox preaching and teaching tradition also affirms that suffering, which comes to human life unwelcomed and uninvited, can be dealt with in a way that transforms us. The heart, mind, and life of a person who suffers may be refined and purified; suffering may indeed be necessary to prepare our souls for the kingdom of God. Viewed from this perspective, being made to suffer may be an expression of the "mercy of God," for only by that suffering are we able to change so as to be fit for God's kingdom. In this sense, suffering may become an instrument for our benefit.

But Orthodoxy also makes a third affirmation, developed as part of the ascetic tradition of monasticism. It is that the deliberate and conscious submission of one's life to duress and suffering can free it from attachment to what distracts it from the true good—communion with God.

Far from being a "religious masochism" that finds enjoyment in suffering itself, this third approach to suffering is undertaken to free life from those things that cause suffering and to open life to its full potential. This approach is based on the tradition of the "suffering Servant" in Old Testament prophecy; on the example of the freely undertaken "emptying" and "humbling" of Christ in his Incarnation; and most of all on the victory of Christ over death, sin, and evil, on the cross. St. Paul says it all in a few brief verses:

> Have this mind among yourselves, which you have in Christ Jesus, who, though he was in the form of God, did not count equality with God a thing to be grasped, but emptied himself, taking the form of a servant, being born in the likeness of men. And being found in human form he humbled himself and became obedient unto death, even death on the cross. Therefore, God has highly exalted him and bestowed on him the name which is above every name. . . . (Philippians 2:5–10)

Thus one inclusive perspective contains the three approaches to suffering concurrently lived, practiced, and taught in the Orthodox Christian tradition: the avoidance of suffering as an evil, the acceptance of involuntary suffering as a trial given for the benefit of one's life in God, and the encouragement of voluntary suffering as a discipline that can lead to true fulfillment.

THE LIMITING OF SUFFERING

An Orthodox priest has eloquently described the pervasiveness of suffering:

> To the old cliché that nothing is certain in life except death and taxation one could add suffering. For suffering is a universal aspect, or more boldly stated, a condition of living. In every person's life there is at least one moment of pain and suffering, even if that moment is the half-forgotten experience of his birth into the world. For the vast majority of humanity, suffering is far more than a distant, shadowy memory. Rather it is an experience either continuous or intermittent to which we are subject at every turn of life, whether expected or unexpected, welcomed or rejected, desired or despised. [It is] an omnipresent fact of human life. . . . [1]

To avoid suffering completely in this life seems therefore a utopian desire. As we saw in Chapter 4, the fallen condition in which we find ourselves means inevitably that suffering in one form or another will be part of every person's life. The first response of the Orthodox church to this reality is to seek to limit suffering, especially involuntary suffering, in human life. Prayer and philanthropy are two major means toward fulfilling this goal.

In principle, suffering should not be the lot of humankind, or for that matter, of all creation. The true cure of suffering is complete restoration of the communion of created existence with God. Because of freedom, and because of the license we give to evil and sin in our lives, and because evil is overcome in each person only in the steps of a cumulative process of growth, the only expectation of total freedom from suffering exists in the heavenly kingdom. So it is that in services associated with the funeral rites the Orthodox church prays: "to the soul of this Your servant (Name), departed this life, do You Yourself, O Lord, give rest in a place of light, in a place of green pasture, in a place of refreshment, from where pain and sorrow and mourning have fled away."[2]

In this life, however, suffering comes to us in many ways. This acknowledgment is expressed most fully in the prayers of the bread-blessing service, usually chanted at the end of a feast-day vesper. Unexpectedly, this litany of petitions for protection from sufferings is found in a service of thanksgiving to God for the multitude of his blessings, which includes prayers that he continue to pour out his material and spiritual blessings upon us. A compilation of passages relating to suffering in this service yields these:

> O Lord our God, who bowed the heavens and came down for the salvation of humanity: Look upon Your servants and Your inheritance. . . . Guard them at all times . . . from every foe, from all adverse powers of the Devil. . . .

> Furthermore we pray . . . for every Christian soul that is afflicted and weary in well-doing, in need of God's mercies and help . . . for the peace and quietness of the whole world; . . . for those who are absent and abroad; for the healing of those who lie in sickness; . . . for the deliverance of captives. . . .

> Furthermore we pray that [God] will preserve this city and this holy Temple, and every city and land from pestilence, famine, earthquake, flood, fire, the sword, the invasion of enemies, and from civil war. . . .

These prayers end with the petition, "hide us under the shadow of Your wings; drive far from us every foe and adversary; make our life peaceful, O Lord. Have mercy upon us and upon Your world; and save our souls, forasmuch as You are gracious and love humankind."[3]

But Orthodoxy has not limited itself to prayer. Philanthropy by Christians of every social rank is also a living practice in the face of human suffering. Every Christian tradition seeks to practice the commandment of Christ's love to those in need. In the great Greek Orthodox Christian empire of Byzantium which existed continuously for over a millennium, a whole range of philanthropic institutions were established by emperors, patriarchs, bishops, monastics, and laypersons. In recent years, historical studies have shown in amazing detail the tremendous geographic spread and wide range of types of philanthropic institutions in Byzantium. Hospitals, hospices, homes for the aged, leprosaria, orphanages, houses for the poor, reformatory homes, cemeteries for the indigent, and homes for the blind existed from the earliest days of the empire, many of which were continued after the fall of the Byzantine Empire, into the period of subjugation to the Muslim Ottoman Empire which followed it in 1453.[4] The impulse to alleviate involuntary suffering is an essential part of Orthodox piety, and these traditions of philanthropy continue, wherever possible, in the Orthodox world today.

THE INEVITABILITY OF SUFFERING

In both prayer and action, Orthodox Christianity recognizes the responsibility to restrict and limit human suffering, but it acknowledges as well that involuntary suffering is frequently unavoidable. In the face of the experience of suffering, it is imperative for the Christian to move beyond the lament that he or she has failed to avoid suffering. Suffering provokes a new attitude from the believer.

This can be illustrated by a commonly conducted service of the Orthodox church, the Sanctification of Waters, in which water is blessed and sprinkled on people and objects so as to sanctify them. This service, perhaps more than any other, brings the sacred into relationship with the ordinary aspects of life. It also incorporates the experience of suffering into the life of the kingdom. The Epistle reading, taken from the New Testament book of Hebrews, focuses on two points: suffering and the sharing of the faithful in Christ's suffering.

> It was fitting that he [God the Father], for whom and by whom all things exist, in bringing many sons to glory, should make the pioneer of their salvation [Jesus Christ] perfect through suffering. For he who sanctifies and those who are sanctified have all one origin. . . . [B]ecause he himself has suffered and been tempted, he is able to help those who are tempted. (Hebrews 2:10–11, 18)

St. John Chrysostom makes some enlightening comments on this passage. While clearly distinguishing between Christ as God and us, God's creatures, Chrysostom also points to the common experience shared by believers and their Lord. Commenting on the phrase "perfect through suffering" and focusing on Christ's sufferings through his Incarnation, he observes: "Then sufferings are a perfecting, and a cause of salvation. Do you see that to suffer affliction is not the portion of those who are utterly forsaken; if indeed it was by this that God first honored His Son, by leading Him through suffering?"[5]

Here is a radical change of attitude; we see something new in suffering. It is more than an evil we seek to avoid. With Chrysostom, we see that in Christ, suffering has a purpose (perfecting), and that it can be a means to salvation. Chrysostom challenges his Christian audience to look upon suffering differently from non-Christians. Instead of seeing suffering as an unmitigated evil (interpreting it as meaning that one has been "utterly forsaken"), Christians can find in it purpose and significance, precisely because it was through suffering that God led Christ into his saving work. Thus "perfecting through suffering" in Christ shows that "suffering for anyone, not only profits 'him' [the person for whom the suffering has taken place], but he himself [Christ] also becomes more glorious and more perfect." What holds true for Christ holds true for the Christian as well. Chrysostom continues, "And this too he says in reference to the faithful, comforting them by the way: for Christ was glorified then when he suffered." Chrysostom proceeds to focus on the sentence "For he who sanctifies and those who are sanctified all have one origin." Again careful not to confuse the divine with the human in any substantive way, he focuses on the communion shared in this experience of suffering. "Behold again how he brings them together, honoring and comforting them, and making them brethren of Christ, in this respect that they are 'of one.' "[6]

The Christian now sees suffering in a new light: it has meaning and purpose for one's ultimate destiny and is shared in a significant way with Christ. This makes the Christian's approach to suffering different from that of nonbelievers. In another place, commenting on St. Paul's description of himself as "sorrowful, yet always rejoicing," Chrysostom discusses the impact of this new attitude toward suffering:

> Now these things he says to instruct us not to be disturbed at the opinions of the many, though they call us deceivers, though they know us not, though they count us condemned, and appointed unto death, to be in sorrow, to be in poverty, to have nothing, to be (us who are in cheerfulness) desponding. . . . For the faithful only are right judges of these

matters, and are not pleased and pained at the same things as other people.[7]

Thus the first step in dealing with suffering from the Christian point of view is a revision of our thought. The Christian's technical term for the change of heart and mind which leads us to see things from the perspective of God, and not from the perspective of our fallen condition, is *repentance*. To speak of repentance here is not at all necessarily to imply moral responsibility for our experience of suffering. To face suffering with repentance is to see suffering as an important means to deeper, more profound growth toward God-likeness. Therefore when suffering comes into our lives uninvited, it becomes a test of faith and Christian living.

SUFFERING AS TRIAL

What is the fundamental nature of the testing that Christians face when they suffer? The monastic and patristic literature describes the trial of suffering in many ways—as a testing of faith, of endurance, of hope, of loyalty, of commitment to the monastic calling. All, however, are subsumed within the fundamental test of discipleship. In facing sufferings we follow either the way of the world or the way of repentance.

If an experience of unwanted suffering leaves us insensitive to the potentialities in it for greater communion with God, then we have faced it not as followers of Christ or as persons who bear the name Christian conscientiously and in practice. If somehow and in some measure we meet involuntary suffering as an opportunity for the refinement of our spirits and growth in God-likeness, then our basic attitude to it is Christian, and we respond as disciples of the Lord.

This does not mean, of course, that we will not be tempted to despair, fear, or hopelessness. It does not mean that we will escape pain and anxiety. It means that the disciple maintains a perspective that incorporates these experiences into the communion he or she lives with God and with his people. St. John Chrysostom exposes the fundamental issue:

> [Jesus] knew so well that tribulation is expedient for us, and that it becomes rather a foundation for repose. For hear Him saying, "If a man take not his cross, and follow after Me, he is not worthy of Me." (Matt. x, 38.) If you are a disciple, He means, imitate the Master; for this is to be a disciple. But if while He went by the path of affliction, you go by the path of ease, you no longer tread on the same path which He trod, but on another. How then do you follow, when you follow not? How shall you be a disciple, not going after the Master?[8]

Chrysostom repudiates the idea that suffering itself might be the cause of our spiritual defeat. Suffering is the occasion for the test, but our failure to respond as disciples is the reason suffering may "overthrow and destroy."

> Affliction does not do this, but our own slothfulness. How, you say? If we are sober and watchful, if we beseech God that He would not "suffer us to be tempted above that which we are able to bear" (I Cor. x. 13), if we always hold fast to Him, we shall stand nobly and set ourselves against our enemy. So long as we have Him for our helper, though temptations blow more violently than all the winds, they will be to us as chaff and a leaf borne lightly along. Hear Paul saying, "In all these things, . . . we are more than conquerors."[9]

Stated another way, the Christian's approach to suffering does not differ from his or her approach to all other aspects of life. Whether we describe the unique Christian way as incarnational, sacramental, ethical, eucharistic, ascetic, eschatological, faithful, spiritual, or redemptive, we are referring to the Christian purpose of realizing God-likeness. This is the fundamental trial. If we fail it, we fall back into the world's way of approaching suffering. Passing it, we enter into the way that is ultimately "approved in Heaven," to use yet another term. So says Chrysostom:

> These things let us take into our mind, beloved, let us consider them, let us hold them in remembrance, and then we shall never faint, though we be wronged, though we be plundered, though we suffer innumerable evils. Let it be granted us to be approved in Heaven, and all things are endurable. Let it be granted us to fare well there, and things here are of no account. These things are a shadow, and a dream; whatever they may be, they are nothing either in nature or in duration, while those are hoped for and expected.[10]

THE TRANSFIGURING POWER OF SUFFERING

It is not suffering itself that transfigures but suffering approached in the spirit of discipleship as an aspect of our growing communion with God. Here we enter a vast area of spiritual experience in the Orthodox religious tradition. Several themes express the transforming power of this fundamental approach in the lives of believers.

The Community of Suffering. In a touching and gentle article on the suffering and death of children, Metropolitan Anthony of Surozh, a contemporary bishop of the Orthodox church in Europe and also a physician, points to the important ecclesial truth that our suffering is rarely if ever limited to ourselves.[11] A Christian will understand the meaning of an experience of suffering not only for the communion of the sufferer and God but for all those who share in it—family, friends, physicians, nurses, social workers, indeed, the cosmos as a whole. We never suffer alone.

Suffering as Witness. After the model of Christ's own suffering comes the suffering of martyrdom. Those in the early church recognized that to suffer persecution was to share in the suffering of the Lord, and they could therefore rejoice in it. The transition from witnessing the faith through bloody martyrdom to witnessing through patient bearing of the sufferings of life was an easy one for the early church. Chrysostom thus says, "It is not only the people dragged into court, those who refused when ordered to make sacrifice, and those who endured suffering who were martyrs, but also those who consented to endure pain for any of God's purposes."[12] To suffer in the spirit of Christ is to make a witness of faith.

The Acceptance of Suffering. Part of the new attitude toward suffering that arises out of committed Christian discipleship is the acceptance of suffering when it comes. The model for this is the ancient canonical approach to martyrdom. The canons of the church condemned those who apostatized when faced with the trial of martyrdom. If challenged by the pagan authorities to deny Christ by offering incense to the gods, the Christian had no alternative but to refuse. On the other hand, the Christian was prohibited from provoking or seeking out martyrdom.[13] The translation to the experience of suffering in the life of the Christian was not at all difficult. Chrysostom puts it, "Even if there be no persecution, nor tribulation, yet there are other afflictions which befall us every day. . . . Let us then pray indeed to God that we may not come into temptation; but if we come into it, let us bear it nobly."[14]

Endurance in Suffering. On the immediate experiential level, the trial of suffering is successfully met when we are able to endure. As we have seen, we will suffer even if we have done nothing deserving of punishment—simply because we live in a fallen world. Accepting that, we endure. "The righteous suffer tribulation here, because they are sojourners, and strangers, and are in a foreign country. The just therefore endure these things for the purpose of trial. . . . Under all circumstances, therefore, whether afflictive or otherwise, let us give thanks to God. For both are beneficial" is Chrysostom's summation in one of his homilies.[15]

The Benefits of Suffering. With the transfiguration of suffering outlined in this chapter, a remarkable perspective comes to the fore in Christian experience. What is originally perceived as an evil to be avoided becomes a means for blessings. As St. Paul put it, "we know that in all things God works for the good of those who love him" (Romans 8:28, New International Version). In the same chapter we have one of the most powerful expressions of Christian response in the face of suffering and tribulation: "What then shall we say in response to this? If God is for us, who can be against us? He who did not spare his own Son, but gave him up for us all—how will he not also, along with him, graciously give us all things" (verses 31–32). It is impossible, here or anywhere, to enumerate "all things" which come to us as a result of faithful endurance of suffering.

At the beginning of his work "Concerning the Statues," St. John Chrysostom provides us with an eight-point list of such consequences "of the diversified and manifold affliction which befalls the saints." He presents them as "reasons" for which God permits his saintly servants to suffer, but they are all consequences of the new experience of suffering that belongs to a follower of the God "who did not spare his own Son." The first is to provide a counterpoint of humility for the "greatness of their good works." The second reason that God permits suffering is so that "others may not have a greater opinion of [the saints] than belongs to human nature." The third is "that the power of God may be made manifest" through "men who are infirm and in bonds." The fourth, "that the endurance of these themselves may become more striking." The fifth good consequence of suffering, according to Chrysostom, is the assurance of the resurrection and life to come given to those who suffer and have not received their reward in this life: "after the end of life here . . . [they] will receive the recompense of the present labors." The sixth is to give "all who fall into adversity . . . a sufficient consolation and alleviation." Another consequence is that Christians may imitate in their lives the virtues of saintly persons. And finally, we can truly understand the nature of life: "that when it is necessary to call any blessed, or the reverse, we may learn whom we ought to account happy, and whom unhappy and wretched."[16]

Voluntary Suffering. As a result, that special class of Christians, the monks, assumed a discipline that removes one's focus from things transitory and brings control over all aspects of one's life, placing that life as much as possible in God's service and in communion with him. The monks counsel the rest of us that some form of this discipline, which they call "voluntary suffering," together with the appropriate acceptance of involuntary suffering, is necessary to all for fulfilling the purpose of human life. This moves us one step further in the comprehensive paradox of the Christian approach to suffering.

Voluntary suffering makes a statement that is difficult for the worldly mind to accept. In the words of St. Peter of Damascus, "Just as sick people need surgery and cautery to recover the health they have lost, so we need trials, and toils of repentance, and fear of death and punishment, so that we may regain our former health of soul and shake off the sickness which our folly has induced." He adds, "The more the Physician of our souls bestows upon us voluntary and involuntary suffering, the more we should thank Him for his compassion and accept the suffering joyfully. . . . In this way, if we voluntarily accept affliction, we will be freed from our sickness and from the punishments to come, and perhaps even from present punishments as well."[17] The paradox is almost complete: if we voluntarily accept suffering, and even impose it on ourselves through freely accepted discipline, we free ourselves of suffering, in this life as well as in the life to come.

Redemptive Suffering. The self-emptying of Christ for the life of the world utterly transforms and turns upside down our perceptions of suffering. Suffering in Christ becomes the occasion for newness of life and salvation. The humiliation he bore transfigures suffering in life into a glory, a manifestation of godliness. What appears to be mere passive acceptance reforms and transfigures the heart of events and makes them into icons of the kingdom, for those who experience them in this self-emptying way.

Russian Orthodoxy perhaps has conveyed this message to the world most fully and deeply through inspired writers like Dostoyevsky. We would go far afield if we entered the vast arena of critical literature that examines these writings.[18] But a summary is provided by an Eastern European Christian quoted in 1982 in an article titled "A Salvation of Suffering: The Church in the Soviet Union." This anonymous Christian accurately reflects the Orthodox perspective:

> You Western Christians often seem to consider material prosperity to be the only sign of God's blessing. On the other hand, you often seem to perceive poverty, discomfort, and suffering as signs of God's disfavor. In some ways we in the East understand suffering from the opposite perspective. We believe that suffering may be a sign of God's favor and trust in the Christian to whom the trial is permitted to come. In one sense it seems to us that God has selected the church in Eastern Europe for a special assignment—suffering. Knowing this, of course, does not mean that our sufferings are not agonizing. But it does provide healing and redemption in our sufferings.[19]

SUFFERING AND THE MEDICAL PROFESSION

Little mention has been made in this chapter of sickness and illness. But what has been said about them in the previous chapter is readily applicable to this more personal and subjective aspect of the same topic. The paradox remains: we are to seek to avoid and heal illnesses; when they come, we are to bear them with fortitude and courage, trusting in God's grace to help us endure; when we are not ill, we are to discipline ourselves and keep our healthy lives fully in communion with God. Suffering in all cases can transform life and become, as an icon experienced, a window opening on heaven.

Hospital chaplains, nurses, physicians, and other health professionals will encounter all these attitudes among Orthodox believers who fall ill. In some cases one or another attitude will dominate; in others they will be in a balance. Not unknown will be what some may characterize as an obdurate willingness to suffer pain and discomfort as "payment for sins." Perhaps the health professional will better understand these Orthodox patients as a result of reading this chapter. Perhaps Orthodox Christians doing the same will not only understand each other better but even deepen their own personal approach to suffering.

Part III
CARING AND CURING

·6·

Human Dignity in Caring
and Curing

The version of the Old Testament considered authoritative in the Orthodox church is the Septuagint, the first translation made of the Hebrew text, which also includes ten books originally written in Greek. Among those ten is Ecclesiasticus, written between 200 and 132 B.C.E.[1] This book contains a passage that summarizes fairly well the mainline approach of the Orthodox church to the sick and their healing:

> My son, in thy sickness be not negligent: but pray to the Lord, and he will make thee whole. Leave off from sin, and order thy hands aright, and cleanse thy heart from all wickedness. Give a sweet savor, and a memorial of fine flour; and make a fat offering, as much as you can afford. Then give place to the physician, for the Lord hath created him: let him not go from thee, for thou hast need of him. There is a time when in their hands there is good success. For they shall also pray unto the Lord, that he would prosper that which they give for ease and remedy to prolong life. He that sinneth before his Maker, let him fall into the hand of the physician![2]

In this passage we see several central themes: the primary reliance on God; the belief that moral, spiritual, and physical health must be considered wholistically; the encouragement of spiritual and liturgical efforts at healing; and the general approval of the medical profession, albeit with some reservations.

What is the foundation for this caring about human well-being and the efforts to cure those who are ill? The Eastern Orthodox tradition points to a certain vision of what it means to be human. The Genesis account of the creation of humanity and the New Testament's pinpointing of the purpose of human life as becoming "God-like" are parts of the same fabric; the purpose of humanity's beginning and end is one. It is this goal and vision that motivates many of our actions toward others, including caring for and seeking to cure the sick.

In this chapter, we will briefly examine this teaching in the Orthodox tradition, trace its application in the concept of philanthropy, consider the question of those thought to be in some way "marginal" or "not normal," and finally draw some conclusions about caring for and curing the sick.

THE IMAGE AND LIKENESS OF GOD

What is it to be a human being? Many in our day see humanity as simply an animal at a higher stage of evolution, with no ultimate purpose. Some come to this view from a materialist philosophy; others are despairing existentialists for whom human life is an absurdity with no meaning. Many define human life in terms of transient values: economics, fame, creativity, family, pleasures, politics, projects, ego, and so on. "I live for my children" is a benign form of this reductionism of the meaning of human existence. Feuerbach's famous dictum "Man is what he eats," Marxism's "homos economicus," and Sartre's "other persons are the enemy" are much more insidious responses to the question.

In contrast to these views is the understanding of human existence in the tradition of Eastern Orthodox Christianity. Humanity is a creation of God. But more than that, humanity is created "in the image and the likeness of God." This biblical teaching is not used merely in a general way to attribute distinction and dignity to human beings. From the earliest period of theological reflection in the Eastern Christian world, the story of humanity's creation was understood in a specific way.

The passage referring to the formation of humanity from dust, and the breathing of life by God so that humanity became a "living soul," immediately creates a distinction between humanity and the rest of the created world. Somewhere in the evolutionary process a unique event took place which qualitatively distinguished humanity from the rest of the animal world. That is both a scientific and a theological statement. For the tradition of revelation, as we have seen, the human being is a composite of body and soul. A disembodied human being, in principle, cannot be conceived. The body is an essential aspect of human existence, hence the Christian doctrine of the resurrection.

Of what does the divine image consist? The first step is to emphasize the definitive aspect of the physical human body. The human body is created not only by the saying of a word as are the other animals: "And God said, 'Let the waters bring forth swarms of living creatures' and . . . 'Let the earth bring forth living creatures according to their kinds . . . ' " (Genesis

1:20, 24). One of the two accounts of the creation of humanity describes God as saying not only "Let us make man" but also "so God created man" (Genesis 1:26, 27). The other account is more explicit: "And God formed man of the dust of the ground and breathed into his nostrils the breath of life, and man became a living soul" (Genesis 2:7). Whatever else these passages might mean for a theological understanding of human existence, they certainly point to the bodily dimension of human life. To be a human being means first to be bodily conceived of human parents. Or in more scientific language, a human being is one who carries the human genetic code in his or her genes.

Yet the body, though essential to what it means to be a human being, is an instrument; it is not the chief bearer of the "image" of God in patristic thought. Rather, the soul or spirit, the "invisible" part of humankind, bears the major thrust of the meaning of the "image of God" in us.

The biblical passage that focuses on the creation of humanity in the "image and likeness of God" has received much attention in the patristic tradition. Referring to the "invisible" part of human nature, the passage has been crucial in helping to define the Orthodox understanding of the meaning of human existence.

The tradition has focused on the biblical description of the *consequence* of humanity's creation in the image of God, which is "dominion." St. Basil puts it dramatically: "First of all He ordained us with the power to rule. O Man, you are a ruling animal!"[3] But it soon became clear that the functioning of this consequence of the image depended on two primary faculties which distinguish humanity from the rest of the material creation and make dominion possible: intelligence and self-determination. Thus St. John of Damascus summarizes the patristic tradition: "the phrase 'after his image' clearly refers to the side of his nature which consists of mind and free will."[4]

Not only do mind and self-determination make possible the exercise of dominion, but, properly understood, they are at the source of all aspects of human existence that precisely characterize the God-likeness of our being. Together they provide us with the potential for the unique phenomena of language, creativity, moral judgment, the sciences and the arts, and education.

Another aspect of human existence often referred to in the patristic literature is the "heart," which includes the other aspects of our humanity. Bishop Kallistos Ware, an Orthodox theologian, defines the heart as the "spiritual centre of man's being, man as made in the image of God, his deepest and truest self. . . . 'Prayer of the heart' means prayer not just of the emotions and affections, but of the whole person, including the body," and, it needs to be added, of the intellect as well.[5] Clearly, the heart goes beyond rationality and self-determining choice. It is precisely the heart that gives "humanity" to many human emotions, to love, virtue, self-evaluation, self-sacrifice, and communication. None of these can exist without the combination of mind and self-determination.

Together, mind, self-determination, and the heart allow for an increase in the genuine quality of life. Part of this quality is communion between each of us and God and among ourselves as fellow human beings, relationships both social and intimate. While the heart cannot exist without the mind and self-determination, the mind and the choosing ability have little "human" content without the heart. And all are intimately related to the reality of our bodily existence.

It is necessary to note that this understanding of human existence is not static. In distinguishing the image from the likeness, the Greek Fathers formulated a dynamic approach to the meaning of human existence. The ancient Hebrew poetic expression was undoubtedly understood as a tautology, as simply a restatement of the same idea in different words. Nonetheless, as early as Origen (185–254 C.E.), who was the first thinker to reflect theologically on the Scriptures, the church began to see in the phrase "the likeness" a dimension of humanity's creation that indicated the need for human cooperation to fulfill God's purpose. "Likeness" meant potential for our fulfillment in God-likeness. So, according to St. Gregory of Nyssa, "On the one hand the 'image' was given to us at creation and with the first moment of our constitution co-exists with us." The "likeness," on the other hand, "is accomplished by means of choice."[6] And St. Basil notes that God "added" this likeness to our self-determining ability, "showing that he places a choice in our self-determining power, which is able to make us become like God."[7]

None of this activity takes place in an individualistic vacuum; it is thoroughly communal and social. Being physically conceived, born, and nurtured is a social act. Being nurtured bodily, intellectually, emotionally, and spiritually is possible only corporately.

To be a human being, then, means to be a fully psychosomatic created being conceived of human parents, endowed with the image of God, and called to realize the potential of the likeness of God in communion with him and with other human beings. Although because of sin we are empirically a distorted and fallen image, and although God's image in us is "corrupted" by evil, the Greek Fathers continuously and forcefully affirmed that we are still an "image of God" whose ultimate purpose is to bring to fruition our divine-likeness, the "likeness of God."

CARING, CURING, AND PHILANTHROPY

The potential for God-likeness gives every person an inviolate dignity that deserves respect. This dignity makes claims upon all of us for each other. Why must we care for our own health and the health of others? Why must we seek to heal ourselves and others of illness? One of the most important characteristics of God-likeness is love: "God is love," we read in 1 John 4:8. The model of full humanity is given by Christ, who united intimately the divine and human natures in his person. Therefore the model of love and the model of caring and curing given by Jesus Christ is a model for full human existence.

Although a large majority of the recorded miracles in the Gospels deals with healing, the healing ministry of Jesus was neither a medical practice nor a campaign to eradicate illness. The miracles were "signs of the kingdom," a means of preaching and manifesting the reality of the new life and existence that was the kingdom of God. The disciples, for example, were sent out "to preach the kingdom and to heal" (Luke 9:2); they were instructed to "heal the sick . . . and say to them, 'the kingdom of God has come near to you' " (Luke 10:9).

In the early church caring for the sick and suffering, regardless of their religious beliefs, nationality, and race soon became a hallmark of the Christian life.[8] Dionysius, the bishop of Alexandria, provides a moving example in his description of the Christian response to a great pestilence that fell upon that city about the year 203:

> The most of our brethren were unsparing in their exceeding love and brotherly kindness. They held fast to each other and visited the sick fearlessly, and ministered to them continually, serving them in Christ. And they died with them most joyfully, taking the affliction of others, and drawing the sickness from their neighbors to themselves and willingly receiving their pains. And many who cared for the sick gave strength to others [and] died themselves having transferred to themselves their death. . . . Truly the best of our brethren departed from life in this manner, including some presbyters and deacons and those of the people who had the highest reputation; so that this form of death, through the great piety and strong faith it exhibited, seemed to lack nothing of martyrdom. . . . But with the heathen everything was quite otherwise. They deserted those who began to be sick, and fled from their dearest friends. And they cast them out into the streets when they were half dead, and left the dead like refuse. . . . [9]

Critical reading of this passage will raise technical questions concerning appropriate methods of care. Theirs was hardly an antiseptic procedure! But nothing will gainsay the quality of love and caring of these early Christians. By the late third and early fourth century Christians were generally substituting the word *philanthropy* for the word *love* or using the terms interchangeably in their speaking, literature, preaching, and hymnody.[10] To be philanthropic was to be God-like.

HUMAN DIGNITY AND THE "MARGINAL PERSON"

We have seen that care for fellow human beings was characteristic of Byzantium, a culture and a society whose soul and spirit *was* Orthodox Christianity. But what of those who lack what is perceived to be the average range of human abilities whether physically or intellectually, or in self-determination? The genetically deficient fetus, the mentally retarded, the mentally and emotionally ill, the alcoholic, the drug addict may fall within this category. So also some would include in the category of the marginal person the elderly who have become incompetent, the terminally ill, even those who are unproductive and "can't do anything." How far down the scale of "humanness" can such people be before they are judged "no longer human" or no longer endowed with the dignity of humanity and worthy of care as human beings?

We will not deal here with the specific bioethical issues raised by all these conditions. Rather, we consider only one question: Can there be a "less than human" level of existence for a being conceived of human parents?

The contemporary response to this question seems to be yes. The determination of who is less than human and therefore not entitled to treatment—to protection of life, for instance—is usually cast in terms of the individual's "normality." Thus, in a contemporary discussion of whether to treat a fetus determined by amniocentesis to be defective, the ethical issue is expressed this way: "Does every fetus have the right to be born, even if that child is going to be deformed or defective? . . . Does every fetus have the right not to be born if it cannot be born healthy and normal?"[11]

It is interesting that the issue is cast in the language of rights, a legal concept. The legal approach does not dominate the Eastern Christian tradition in any area, including this one. "Normal humanity" in the Orthodox tradition is God-likeness. Those who approach this norm are the saints, but all of us are on a continuum of being "less than human." Full humanity includes not only the *donatum* of intelligence, self-determination, heart, and all that comes with them, but also growth in the "likeness."

Consequently, falling within the range of some IQ score judged "average" does not necessarily make us more human than a person who doesn't reach that score. Nor does having a score higher than the average make us "more human." The combination of human body, mind, self-determination, and heart in the Orthodox understanding of the "image" means that *what* we do with whatever level of "humanity" we are given is a much greater determinant of our humanity than the rating of our level of intelligence or any other quantitatively measurable characteristic. Those unquantifiable dimensions of human life—love and caring, appreciation of beauty, moral sensitivity, spirituality—may indicate more of one's humanity than raw intellect.

Yet the point is this. All individuals conceived of human parents possess an intrinsic worth, based on what they *are* and what they are *called to be* rather than on what they can accomplish or achieve or contribute. Focusing on the mentally retarded, but applicable to all those who might be considered "marginal" human beings, these words seem appropriate from an Eastern Christian perspective:

> Those who measure human worth in terms of usefulness and cost effectiveness alone see no conflict in treating the retarded, the poor, the imprisoned, the aged as objects—not as persons. But over and over again, persons who are mentally retarded prove to us that even the most handicapped, the least powerful, the most vulnerable . . . (when measured in dollars and cents) have an intrinsic humanity that must be respected and have gifts of character that must be treasured. In our treatment of mentally retarded persons we have a commitment to equality of treatment, to respect, to justice, to the intrinsic worth of every human life.[12]

From an Eastern Orthodox perspective this intrinsic worth emerges from the understanding of humanity as having the potential for God-likeness. It is that potential, never fulfilled in this earthly existence, always open to both a measure of distortion and a measure of fulfillment, which makes us human.

Many issues remain unresolved by this perspective; they require analysis, study, and investigation. This perspective does, however, accord to every human being a status of existence that has meaning, purpose, intrinsic value, and significance. Because of that, we must care for ourselves and for others. No human life is without worth; no human existence is deserving of abandonment. A moral imperative arises in the face of the human worth located in our creation "in the image and likeness of God." We *must* respond to that intrinsic human value in every person with care and concern. Responding selflessly to the needs of our fellows, especially the most weak and defenseless, is the essence of the love shown by Jesus Christ to be at the heart of God-like behavior. In short, to be truly human we must be fundamentally *philanthropic*, literally "loving humanity" in every human being, even the most "marginal."

HUMAN DIGNITY AND MENTAL ILLNESS

Concern for the mentally ill, one group of "marginal persons," appears early in the Christian tradition in Christ's healing of the "demon-possessed."

In these healings Jesus is usually described by the Gospels as simply ordering the demonic power to depart, so that healing may take place. It became traditional in the liturgical life of the Eastern Orthodox church to address these and similar intractable conditions with prayers of exorcism. The symptoms of possession are wide ranging in these prayers. In an exorcism attributed to St. Basil, God is called upon to turn away from the soul of the afflicted person

> every infirmity, every faithlessness, every spirit which is unclean, distressful . . . greedy, prideful, lustful . . . impudent. Yes, Lord, turn away from your servant every activity of the devil, every magical action, every poison, idolatry, witchery, astrology, necromancy, divination, . . . drunkenness, whoring, adultery, lewdness, . . . anger, contentiousness, disorder, and every evil inclination.

The interconnectedness of physical, emotional, moral, intellectual, and spiritual dimensions is evident. But symptoms of mental illness are also specifically included in the exorcisms. Thus, in an exorcism attributed to St. John Chrysostom, the demonic is described as "harming and altering the mind of man."[13]

In the exorcisms the method for removing the offending demonic influence is a command based on the name, the power, and the saving work of God in Christ and the Holy Spirit. In one prayer, for example, the demonic powers are exhorted to "depart from the servant of God (name), from the mind, from the soul, from the heart, from the kidneys, from the senses, from all the members, so that he may be healthy and whole and free, to know his own Lord and the Creator of all, God. . . . "[14] The wholistic perspective is clearly articulated here.

Until the advent of some modern therapies, little beyond such prayers could be done to assist the mentally ill. Whatever else it meant or accomplished, recourse to the exorcism was and still is evidence that the "marginal humanity" of the mentally ill person is not ignored or placed beyond the concern of the religious community. Evidence now being collected indicates that the coherence of mental, physical, moral, and spiritual health continued to be a principle of concern among the Orthodox who sought healing for the mentally ill in the post-Byzantine period.[15]

Historically speaking, the Orthodox had very little involvement in developing modern psychological therapeutic approaches to mental illness. It is important to note that modern psychology and psychiatry arose in the West and tended to focus on a set of perceptions of the human condition rooted in a Western mind-set. For example, one could note that *guilt*, which holds an extremely important place in Freudianism, is a concept highly dependent upon a dominantly legal understanding of life. The East, of course, did not draw so strongly on legal perspectives in interpreting the meaning and values of life. Though guilt was certainly not absent from its worldview, it was not as central as it was in the West. As we saw in the first chapters of this book, relationship was a more controlling perspective in Eastern Christendom. This does not mean, however, that Orthodoxy today holds a uniform attitude toward psychology.

The mainline contemporary Orthodox perspective on modern psychological and psychiatric treatment methods is essentially appreciative, but dissenting voices are heard as well. Three general perspectives coexist. On one extreme is the view that modern psychology itself is demonic and is an essential denial of Orthodox truth. Insofar as much contemporary psychological theory is predominantly atheistic, antireligious, and morally relativistic, this view is justified. In its rejection of all the insights and accomplishments of contemporary psychological theory and practice, however, this first view does not represent the mainline Eastern Orthodox perspective, which is rooted in an appreciation for science and knowledge of the created world.[16]

The mainline view approaches modern psychology critically from the perspective of Orthodox Christian truth and theology. It tends to be positive, discounting the clearly antithetical views, and finds connections between the psychological insights of the church fathers and the approaches developed by some modern schools of psychological therapy.[17]

Even more appreciative of the modern psychological and psychiatric disciplines is the work, in Greece, of such Orthodox Christian psychiatrists as A. A. Aspiotes. Spiritually and religiously based, the Institute of Medical

Psychology and Mental Health under Aspiotes did ground-breaking work in establishing psychological understandings and therapies in Greece during the 1950s and 1960s. His work *Sickness and the Soul* (in Greek) was followed by forty-eight more publications of the institute on various topics of scientific psychological interest.[18]

Yet even as there is appreciation for the development of the sciences of psychology and psychiatry, the Orthodox church maintains trust in its own healing methods as well. It holds that fullness of health requires more than the theories and practices that the world supplies. In its spiritual efforts at healing, the church believes that God acts and that his presence heals. Metropolitan Anthony of Surozh, mentioned above, has reflected on this dimension of the church's healing ministry:

> Apart from any psychological understanding, apart from any intellectual or emotional response, a living soul meets the living God: and the sacraments of the Church address themselves to this living soul which does *not* depend for its knowledge of God on intelligence, consciousness and so on.
>
> But if this is true, then it applies also to all those other things that happen in the body or soul of a child, before the moment it can be intellectually aware of what is happening. As far as grown-ups are concerned, I think, from what I have seen, that it applies to people who are mentally ill, who are beyond reach, who seem to be completely separated from the surrounding world, and who may recover, and whom we meet no longer where we left them, but as men and women who have matured and become greater than they were, as though behind this screen of folly, of madness, the life of the Spirit has continued, because God cannot be stopped or kept out by what is going on in our intellect. God has direct access. God meets a human at the level of his soul that is ultimately the level of silence, of those things which are beyond words; at the level of mystery, of those things which can be known within the silence, but which cannot be expressed by words otherwise than symbolically.[19]

This guiding principle finally determines the approach of Eastern Christianity to those who in one way or another appear to many as "marginally human" or as "no longer human." The first may well characterize nearly all of us; the latter may never be said of one conceived of human parents. Whatever problems this may cause in the area of medical technology and bioethics, the fundamental affirmation of the Orthodox tradition is that essential human dignity is an inalienable divine gift. In some way everyone conceived of human parents is a human being, with more or fewer gifts of the divine image, and more or less realization of the likeness of God.

· 7 ·

Doctors, Priests, and Rational Medicine

Those called to minister to the needs of others inevitably must address human illness. Sickness comes to all of us, sooner or later. That the care of the sick is the business of physicians is self-evident. But what of the church and its pastoral ministrations? It should not surprise anyone that the Orthodox church should have recourse to such spiritual means of healing the sick as prayer, sacraments, and an appeal to saints. What may surprise contemporary people is that in the almost-two-thousand-year history of Eastern Orthodox Christianity, there is also an important place among the concerns of the church for what we may call rational medicine.

By *rational medicine* I mean an approach to healing that rests on an accumulated knowledge of diagnosing and healing human illnesses in a disciplined and organized way. This method uses observation, medications, and surgical procedures and is part of a tradition of healing exercised since ancient times by the medical profession. I distinguish this *rational medicine* from its contemporary development, *scientific medicine,* whose methods since the early nineteenth century have so outstripped the achievements of rational medicine that it must be seen, though in continuity with its predecessor, as radically superior and qualitatively different.

Both rational medicine and scientific medicine nevertheless are distinguished from religious faith and ordinary religious practices. And rightly so. But much evidence shows that in Orthodox Christianity rational medicine and scientific medicine have not been generally perceived as antithetical to religious belief and practice. Rather, the opposite is true.

History demonstrates a remarkably close relationship between rational medicine and Orthodox Christian religious belief and practice throughout the centuries. In the background of this intimate relationship is the early church's general approach to culture and science, and in particular to medicine.

69

CULTURE, SCIENCE, MEDICINE, AND THE CHURCH

From the beginning of the Christian era, as the church came into contact with the Greco-Roman world, it established and maintained a paradoxical relationship toward it. Scholars have searched the Scriptures and the patristic tradition and found at least three approaches toward the "world" and its values. One view has emphasized the contrasts between the life of faith and the values of the world. Thus Tertullian (160–220 C.E.) asks the famous question "What indeed has Athens to do with Jerusalem?" fully expecting a negative answer.[1] This view drew a sharp line between the Christian truth on the one hand and what was viewed as the distorted and valueless pronouncements of the unenlightened philosophers and purveyors of "false knowledge" on the other. This was always a minority view in the church.

Very few voices within the church were willing to go to the other extreme: exalting secular philosophical truth above the pronouncements of the Orthodox faith. Those who did were almost universally condemned as teaching heresy. Such were the Gnostics of the early church whose regard for the Neoplatonist philosophers was so high that they reinterpreted the plain teachings of Scriptures and transformed the faith of the church into a fantastic worldview. These teachings were readily exposed and condemned by early church fathers like Irenaeus, the bishop of Lyons (130–220).[2]

The third attitude to worldly knowledge, science, and culture was the mainline approach of three Eastern church fathers from the province of Cappadocia of Asia Minor—St. Basil the Great, St. Gregory of Nazianzus, and St. Gregory of Nyssa—and St. John Chrysostom. Their view came to represent the central teaching of the church and thus informed the whole mind-set of Byzantium. The Cappadocians, "three brilliant leaders of philosophical Christian orthodoxy in the later 4th century,"[3] appreciated culture, reason, and science and found no major problem in using them when they did not conflict with foundational Christian doctrines.

Their approach to these aspects of human experience was essentially eclectic. For example, St. Basil (c. 330–379) counseled that the education of young Christians should reject what was false and harmful according to the Christian faith and embrace as valuable and appropriate all the rest. One sphere of knowledge most readily adopted was the rational medicine of the epoch. St. Gregory of Nazianzus (329–389) and St. Gregory of Nyssa (330–395) were equally appreciative of the contributions of rational medicine. Gregory, bishop of Nyssa, made significant references to many aspects of medicine known in his day: clinical medicine, physicians, pathology, therapeutic methods—including the use of drugs, medications, and surgery. He described the physician as attending to ills of both body and spirit (that is, the whole person) and thought that demonic origins of illness were to be diagnosed only in unusual circumstances.[4]

Yet such affirmations—given the background out of which these and other church fathers spoke—could not be unequivocal. Medicine, in the mind of the church, was one of the many disciplines not based on divine revelation. Nevertheless, it could not stand as autonomous or completely distinct from the source of truth, who is God; the spiritual would always have precedence. Darrel W. Amundsen, a historian of the patristic approach to medicine, summarizes this attitude:

> Medicines and the skill of physicians are blessings from God. It is not *eo ipso* wrong for a Christian to employ them, but it is sinful to put one's faith in them entirely since, when they are effective, it is only because their efficacy comes from God who can heal without them. Thus to resort to physicians without first placing one's trust in God is both foolish and sinful. Likewise to reject medicine and the medical arts entirely is not only not recommended but is disparaged.[5]

In their writings some of the Byzantine church fathers emphasized the discontinuity between faith and nonrevelatory knowledge, asserting the transcendence of faith, while others focused on the communion and continuity of faith and worldly knowledge.[6] Nevertheless, in general Orthodox Christians in Byzantium held faith truths and scientific truths together in a single perspective. This merging of the spiritual dimensions of life and the nonrevelatory dimensions characterized most of the main expressions of culture in Byzantium. An example is the perception of the relationship of church and state as two aspects of a single reality, expressed in the characteristic term *symphonia*. According to this view, both the emperor and the patriarch served the one people, who were also the people of God. Neither was in theory subject to the other, but both were united in common faith and shared service; each was responsible for different aspects of the life of the people.[7] A similar view was taken of the relationship of human health to rational medicine and spiritual healing. Rational medicine proved to be very important for the church, but it fit into a larger pattern. On the one hand, medicine would not be confused with the traditions of spiritual healing; but on the other, medicine would not be sharply divided from spiritual healing. This, too, was a dimension of faith not only to be taught and proclaimed but to be put into practice.

RATIONAL MEDICINE IN ORTHODOX ENVIRONMENTS

How did rational medicine fare in the historic environments of the Orthodox Christian tradition? Was this science suppressed, or did it flourish? Given the tremendous importance of the Orthodox church for the public and social life of one of its most representative periods—the Byzantine— this is a significant question.

Until a short time ago, the standard histories of medicine published in the non-Orthodox West asserted that rational medicine did not fare well in Byzantium.

> Among medical historians, the commonly held opinion of Byzantine medicine is one of stagnation, plagiarism of the great medical figures of classical antiquity, and a somber boredom that seemingly awaited the Italian Renaissance. . . . Typical is Majno's " . . . after Galen, the history [of medicine] grinds to a halt for at least one thousand years."[8]

Medical historian John Scarborough's recent ground-breaking work on Byzantine medicine counters this negative assessment. He cites the work of "a slowly growing number of scholars" who have challenged "this Gibbonesque attitude toward the medicine of a millennium, in one of the great civilizations of history." Before describing this new view of medicine in Byzantium, however, a disclaimer must be made. Nothing in Eastern (or Western) Christendom's pre-nineteenth-century history compares with the advances of science and medicine in the modern period, and we need to be careful not to overstate the achievements of Byzantine medicine as its story is being corrected.

The new range of studies in the history of medicine does indicate that Byzantine rational medicine was remarkably developed. Previously unexamined historical documents witness to a rational medicine significantly more advanced than that which existed in Western Christendom during the twelve-hundred-year existence of what historian Arnold Toynbee has called the "Orthodox Christian Civilization" of Byzantium.[9] Thus, even after all the qualifying statements have been made, medical historian John Scarborough's general assessment of rational medicine in Byzantium is impressive:

> Literary sources . . . verify the typical pre-supposition of a sophisticated medical knowledge, widely diffused among the upper strata of the Byzantine Empire; such medicine was practiced by skilled professionals, well schooled in the theory of medicine. . . .

The medical sources also disclose a lively and constant activity. Old traditions and fresh observations are reworked, recombined, and reorganized according to the shifting needs of Byzantine society.[10]

Many papers in the Dumbarton Oaks *Symposium on Byzantine Medicine* deal with the relationship of medicine and religion; others rely on religiously oriented writings which both directly and indirectly provide evidence of the state of the discipline of medicine. One article discusses the methods of Byzantine medical education, including the time-honored method of apprenticeship as well as structured study at medical schools. A full description is given of one of Byzantium's best-known physicians, Alexander of Tralles, who based his work not only on the writings of the ancients but on his own experience and observations, which he recorded near the end of his life in a therapeutic handbook for the benefit of other physicians.[11]

THE BYZANTINE HOSPITAL AND THE ORTHODOX CHURCH

Throughout the history of Byzantium a minority voice minimized the value of rational medicine, preferring to trust only in God and his saints for healing. Nevertheless, this was not true of the mainline practice and teaching in the church.

Generally speaking, rational medicine found a hospitable environment in Byzantium: the state apparatus provided support, protection, and regulation,[12] and the church also gave support. Not only did well-known church fathers speak favorably of physicians and their medical art, but many were fond of using medical analogies for the spiritual work of the church. Early in the history of the church, Clement of Alexandria (150–215) uses the metaphor of the physician to describe Christ, and with him the Christian patristic tradition assumed a similar perspective: "the Word of the Father, who made man, cares for the whole nature of His creature; the all-sufficient Physician of humanity, the Saviour, heals both body and soul."[13]

The Fathers also compared medical methods for healing the body to spiritual methods for healing the soul. The many analogies they found indicate their acceptance and approval of medical practice. Thus Chrysostom, speaking of the need to change the patterns of sinful living, argued: "For the physicians too give us directions to cure contraries by contraries. Is fever, for instance, produced by a full diet? They subject the disease to the regimen of abstinence. . . . Thus also it befits us to act, with respect to the diseases of the soul."[14]

But the church's confidence in rational medicine transcended literary devices and words of approbation. It was the Orthodox church that provoked the organization of the medical profession for the systematic care and healing of patients in the hospital setting. Church leaders not only spoke well of physicians but employed them in a hitherto unknown way to implement the church's philanthropic goals. The Byzantine hospital is the strongest evidence of a wholesome and healthy cooperative relationship between the Orthodox Christian tradition and rational medicine.

In 1985 Timothy S. Miller published *The Birth of the Hospital in the Byzantine Empire*, which illuminated the positive relationship between the Eastern Orthodox Christian tradition and rational medicine as a discipline.[15] The title might be understood to denote a regional study of hospitals within Byzantium, a companion volume among others on the history of hospitals in France, Germany, Italy, and England, for example. But that is not the case: Miller shows that the very institution of the hospital was born and flourished in Byzantium.

Technically speaking, a hospital is not a place where sick people are gathered so that they may be comforted in their suffering. Such institutions existed for many centuries in both the East and the West. According to Miller, a hospital is an "institution which provides beds, meals, and constant nursing care for its patients while they undergo medical therapy at the hands of professional physicians. It was not until the eighteenth century that anything approaching that definition existed in the West in any significant way." Miller contends that "with the exception of a seventh-century example in Visigoth Spain, none of the philanthropic institutions of Western Europe seem to have offered the sick access to professional physicians before the twelfth century." Even so, "researchers have emphasized that hospitals of the medieval West fell so short of modern notions of proper patient care that they cannot be considered true forefathers of twentieth-century medical centers."[16]

In contrast, Miller piles up evidence showing that the ancestors of the modern hospital are to be found in Byzantium, beginning as early as the fourth century. These places of healing were originally expressions of Christian philanthropy for the poor and for strangers (hence their original name *xenones*, meaning "places for strangers"). It was for the medical care of the sick in these institutions that the church of the Eastern Roman Empire (that is, Byzantium) engaged private physicians, organized them, financed them, and thus gave birth to the hospital in history.

Thus, the Byzantine *xenones* represent not only the first public institutions to offer medical care to the sick, but also the mainstream of hospital development through the Middle Ages, from which both the Latin West and the Moslem East adopted their facilities for the ill. *To trace the birth and development of centers for the sick in the Byzantine Empire is thus to write the first chapter in the history of the Hospital itself.*[17]

It is critical to note that it was the church in the East that established the *xenones* and the hospitals, or *nosokomeia* (literally, "places for the care of the sick"). The church governed the hospitals, financed them, and provided their staffing. It did this as an expression of its Christian calling to "love humanity" and as an embodiment of its calling to become God-like; God was above all *philanthropos,* "one who loves humanity." Thus, after mentioning the "significant roles" of the Cappadocians and Chrysostom in the early years of Christian hospitals, Miller expresses in general terms the intimate relation between the Orthodox church and the development of the hospital.

> As the orthodox church came to exalt the medical profession as the epit-ome of philanthropia, it in turn felt obliged to make this philanthropia available to all—especially the poor—by sponsoring hospitals. Since most Greek church leaders continued to esteem medicine as one of the best expressions of Christian love until the final days of the East Roman Empire, so too they did not falter in supporting nosokomeia. As late as the 1440's the monastery of John Prodromos in Petra still maintained a public hospital.[18]

As this quotation indicates, hospitals in Byzantium were frequently part of monastic establishments. The founding charters of many monasteries in-cluded provisions and rules of governance for these hospitals for the gen-eral public (which were in addition to the infirmaries devoted to the exclusive treatment of the monks). One of the most famous was the hospi-tal in the twelfth-century Pantokrator Monastery whose charter (*typikon*) shows a highly professional organization, with administration in the hands of the monastics, the medical care and surgery handled by carefully graded staffs of physicians, and ranks of supportive staff drawn from the monastics. The hospital had specialized clinics and the necessary physical facilities to fulfill its tasks.[19]

MODERN ORTHODOXY AND MEDICINE

The compatibility between Orthodoxy and rational medicine remained in the Orthodox world even after the dissolution of the Byzantine Empire, though not quite in the same way in Orthodox Russia. There, Tsar Peter the Great drew primarily on the developing science of medicine in the West to develop Russian institutions of medical science and healing. Nevertheless, it was clergy who sent their sons and daughters to the new medical schools to become physicians with a frequency highly disproportionate to their numbers in the population. This indirectly indicates a sense of compatibility between faith and rational medicine, even though part of the motive was certainly the desire to advance socially and economically.[20]

At this same time, within the Muslim Ottoman Empire, which had ended the political existence of Byzantium in 1453, the Orthodox were seriously limited in their ability to continue the tradition of intimate relationship between faith and medicine because of the strictures of their second-class citizenship. Nevertheless, significant steps were taken to provide for medical care. It was Christians, by and large, who became physicians for both the Muslim overlords and the subject Christian peoples, since the Turks felt it was beneath their dignity to do such "menial work." Young Orthodox Christian men usually studied at the renowned medical schools in Italy and returned to influential practices within the Ottoman Empire. Medicine offered Orthodox Christians a promising career; it provided not only material rewards but a significant measure of influence.[21]

Among these Orthodox physicians were the especially distinguished "physician-philosophers" (Greek, *iatrophilosophoi*). The physician-philosophers were distinguished from other physicians by their interest in theology and by their reverence and piety. An example was Eustratios Argenti (1687–1757), who practiced medicine and wrote theology on the island of Chios. He proudly identified himself in his books as an *iatrophilosophos*.[22] To this day, many Orthodox Christian physicians find no conflict in relating their profession as medical doctors with spiritual and religious interests, even on an academic level. An example is John Papavasiliou, a practicing physician and member of the faculty of the Medical School of the University of Athens. In his article "Modern Biology and Christian Faith" he relates scientific understandings of the "microbial world" and bioethical and spiritual questions. He holds that "the new developments of Biology must be taken into consideration by Religion, at least because of their biomedical implications and their importance for Christian sociology (i.e. social ethics) and morality." He also discusses "the Bible, science, and evolution," taking a standard Orthodox stance between a mechanistic view and a literalist perspective on creation. His article concludes with a theological section: "Life, Death and Resurrection."[23]

Nor did the tradition of Christian hospitals die out during the Ottoman period. The church and the medical profession cooperated in establishing the first Christian hospital in the Ottoman Empire in 1517, sixty-four years after the fall of Constantinople. Others were established in the patriarchates of Alexandria and Jerusalem. Nearly all were associated with monasteries as was the traditional practice. Often these hospitals were located in provincial locales, not only in major cities.[24]

What of contemporary attitudes? In 1985 I solicited the opinions of Greek Orthodox physicians regarding the relationship between medicine and religion among their Greek Orthodox patients.[25] Several physicians clearly indicated that they saw no conflicts between religion and their medical practice with Greek Orthodox patients. One physician observed, "I have found that religion and medicine can work together to help a patient reach good mental and physical health." Together with a number of other physicians, he observed that "many patients with 'difficult' medical problems do better than expected because of their faith." One physician enthusiastically extolled the power of faith in healing: "[I] enunciate to patients that FAITH is our survival kit; and that, truly, it 'moves mountains!' The positive attitude and FAITH are protective." This of course applies to religious faith in general, not only to the Orthodox. In this same general perspective, another doctor remarked that the "positive aspects of religious belief are most clearly seen in patients with severe medical problems. Strong faith, under those circumstances, can be of great help to the patient in distress. Such faith, by the way, is not dissimilar to what I have observed among other Christians." Another physician observed, "I cannot remember even one objection based on religious grounds being made about a medical recommendation of mine."

Some conflicts were recognized, however. One blamed these conflicts on "illiterate and stupid and fanatic clergymen in Greece," and a few others made similar comments. On the other side, another physician commented that a clergyman was particularly helpful to him in dealing with a case regarding the continuation or cessation of life-support procedures. The church's opposition to abortion was highlighted most frequently, especially in connection with thalassemia, or Cooley's anemia, which is met in significant proportion among Greek Orthodox people. An inherited blood disease which causes death in its victims by their mid-twenties, thalassemia can be detected *in utero*. Other topics mentioned were decision making on the continuation of life support systems, permission for an autopsy (which some Orthodox consider a desecration of the mortal remains), and an emphasis on seeking forgiveness of sins rather than healing (reflecting the view that illnesses are "sin-specific"). But the general impression from the physicians' responses was that conflicts between the Orthodox faith and the practice of medicine were minimal.

Since 1980, efforts have been made at an Orthodox institution of higher education in the United States to relate the concerns of medicine, psychology and religion. Because of the high incidence of thalassemia among the Greek Orthodox, one of the earliest efforts was a symposium on that disease held at Hellenic College–Holy Cross Greek Orthodox School of Theology, Brookline, Massachusetts, in March 1985. The symposium brought together physicians, psychologists, theologians, social workers, and leaders of thalassemia-related organizations.[26]

In 1986 the Orthodox Christian Association of Medicine, Psychology and Religion was organized, bringing together physicians, psychologists, and persons primarily concerned with Orthodox Christianity to deal with areas of common interest. Among its stated goals was to "work towards an understanding of the whole person, integrating the basic assumptions of medicine, psychology and religion and the Orthodox Christian faith."[27] The organization, known by its acronym OCAMPR, has struck a responsive chord among Orthodox Christians of many different Orthodox jurisdictions in the U.S. and Canada, and eight organized districts now exist in the U.S. Such organized efforts testify that there is no essential conflict between medicine, the helping professions, and Orthodox Christian religious conviction.

Greek theologian Megas Farantos has traced the history of the conflict between the physical sciences and theology over the past several centuries. He concludes that in principle, from an Orthodox Christian perspective, science and theology are not in fundamental conflict but that they "mutually complement and fulfill each other":

> Science examines the particular and gives great importance to the objective. Theology, with its starting point and center in God as the reality and power which determines all things, seeks to bring humanity as a whole into relationship with the world as a whole, and into contact with its many facets. For only that person who elevates the particular reality and the particular purposes of life into a connection to the whole and ultimate purpose of his or her life and that of the whole world understands the world correctly and lives in full consciousness. . . .
> . . . At their heart, they in fact mutually complement and fulfill each other. Science gives to theology the concrete and the objective, while theology gives to science an inclusive perspective of the reality of the cosmos, especially in its subjective resonances.[28]

· 8 ·
Spiritual Healing: The Saints

Somewhere between a total reliance on rational medicine and an understanding of illness as the direct consequence of demonic influences lies the main realm of the Orthodox church's involvement with the curing of illness. A good name for it is "spiritual healing." In this realm the saints and the liturgical life of the church play important roles. For most people, it is precisely in these two areas that the domain of the church and the need for healing and curing meet. This chapter surveys the saints as healers, and Chapter 9 discusses the liturgical tradition of healing in Orthodoxy. Because of its central importance, however, the sacrament of healing, that is, holy unction, will be considered separately, in Chapter 10.

A TRANSITIONAL FIGURE: THE CLERGY-PHYSICIAN

A transitional figure in the Orthodox tradition is the clergy-physician, who represents a clear acceptance of rational medicine but whose main focus and identity is spiritual and religious rather than scientific. These clergy-physicians, both priests and bishops, embody in their lives the long history of a church that locates in first place the healing power of God, and secondarily, the ministrations of the physician and rational medicine, yet sees them in essential harmony. This universal tradition of the church was represented by Fathers like Gregory of Nazianzus in the East and Jerome and Augustine in the West.[1]

The tradition of the clergy-physician brought together in the same person and in an unforced manner the practice of rational medicine and spiritual healing. Uniting the two concerns was a disposition of "sympathy and reverence before the evils suffered by others," in the words of sixth-century patriarch John the Faster.[2] Tradition held that "Luke the beloved physician" mentioned in Colossians 4:14 was identical with the Evangelist. The canonical Gospel bearing his name, as well as the book of the Acts of the Apostles, bears literary evidence of his dual calling. He became a paradigm for Byzantine physicians generally, and clergy-physicians in particular.

79

A number of clergy-physicians have been identified in the history of the Orthodox church.[3] For example, two early figures were bishops: Theodotus, bishop of Laodicea, who participated in the First Ecumenical Council; and Zenobius of Aegis in Cilicia, who lived under Emperor Diocletian and who also attended the Council of Nicea. As a physician the latter is described as having given free medical care to the poor, while concurrently functioning as a bishop of his people. Though there were some exceptions, it appears that most clergy-physicians became so when, as already practicing physicians, they were ordained.

We know that this was a continuing tradition in Byzantium because as late as the twelfth century, an official effort was made to curtail the practice. Yet it seems not to have succeeded:

> Patriarch Lukas Chrysoberges (1157–1169/70), issued an encyclical precluding deacons and priests trained in the medical profession from practicing medicine along with their religious ministry and other clergy from studying and later practicing medicine. He considered it improper for persons of the cloth to change into medical robes and associate with physicians. Despite the patriarch's ruling, it is doubtful whether physicians were excluded from the priesthood.[4]

The institution of the clergy-physician has survived into the modern period. Two leading physicians of Greece, before and soon after its liberation from the Ottoman Empire, Parthenios Petrakes and Dionysios Pyrros, were priests. In 1812 Pyrros established the first scientific school in Athens and became the first president of the Medical Society of newly liberated Greece.[5] A contemporary example is Metropolitan Anthony of Surozh, mentioned previously, who was a practicing physician before being ordained to the priesthood. There are scattered today among the various Orthodox jurisdictions in the U.S. a few clergy-physicians, though they are far from typical in today's church. Nevertheless, the figure of a clergy-physician was still authentic enough in 1984 to be included in *I, Giorgios*, by William J. Lederer (author of *The Ugly American*). In this novel, which takes place in contemporary Greece and deals with issues of the "inner life," a significant figure interacting with the protagonist is a bishop-physician. The following conversation between them emphasizes the theme of the wholeness of health:

> I asked him, "How is it that you, a bishop, are also a physician?"
> "Long ago," he said, taking the stethoscope from his ears for a few moments, "I felt that the body, the mind, and the spirit each are separate entities and yet, still, they are one—just like the Holy Trinity. Each

is equally sacred and each requires equal attention. If one of them gets polluted or sick, then the others also malfunction; and as we're made in the image of God, every part of us must be as healthy as possible or we are an insult to God. So I decided that if I were to be a priest, I would have to know as much about the body and the mind as I knew about the spirit. I studied the body at medical school. . . . "

"Heidelberg," said Maria [the bishop-physician's sister], smiling proudly.

"I studied the mind with a psychiatrist."

"Doctor Carl Jung," said Maria.[6]

If treated not as a theological text but as the expression of an outlook, the passage succeeds in capturing the underlying rationale that justified the tradition of the clergy-physician.

Nevertheless, it was not the clergy-physician who captured the imagination and devotion of the faithful in uniting medicine and faith. Rather, the saint-physician assumed that role.

THE UNMERCENARY SAINT-PHYSICIANS

Among the "nine orders of saints," such as the apostles, martyrs, confessors, and Fathers of the Church, is found the class of the "unmercenary saint-physicians" (the holy *anargyroi*, literally, the "silverless" saints). *The Priest's Service Book* mentions several of these "wonder-working Unmercenaries": Kosmas and Damian, Kyros and Ioannes, Sampson and Diomedes, Mokius and Akinatus, Thalalaius, Hermolaus, and Panteleimon.[7] All these saints seem to have had some kind of medical training. One of the most popular was St. Panteleimon, martyred under Emperor Maximian about the year 305, according to tradition. It is believed that he was born in Nicomedeia, a city in the northern part of Asia Minor, near the Black Sea. As a youth he bore the name Pantoleon. His father, Eustorgius, was a pagan, while his mother, Euboula, was born into a Christian family. It was she who encouraged him to become a Christian, which he did under the tutelage of the priest Hermolaus.

Panteleimon had studied medicine under the well-known physician Euphrosynus and was well-known for the healing art when he was baptized. He quickly obtained the reputation of an "unmercenary healer," a man of philanthropy toward the poor. The traditional story of the saint's martyrdom incorporates the healing dimension of his ministry. The saint is credited with healing a blind man, but when the healing comes to the attention of the emperor, he first kills the man who has been healed and then brings martyrdom to the saint by torturing him and finally having his head cut off. One of the hymns of his feast, held annually on July 27, characteristically expresses the pious expectations of the faithful: "Streams of grace and healing freely flow forth as from a great fountain upon all that seek for the aid of Panteleimon, the godly-wise physician. Come, therefore, ye that thirst for strength and health, be ye filled." As a healer, he is "an imitator of the Merciful One," but his powers are not his own, for he is "one who received from Him [Christ] the grace of healing."[8]

The physician-saints are readily available to heal those who suffer from illnesses. As with many classes of saints, their hymns have become formalized and repeat similar phrases; they give evidence of a coherent attitude. Those of Sts. Kosmas and Damian, who are commemorated on November 1 each year, serve as an example:

> Living humbly on earth, . . . you were granted great gifts! Going everywhere to heal the sick . . . heal now our sufferings.
>
> You kept the purity of your souls stainless, opposing material desires . . . you require no gold when healing the sick. . . .
>
> With Christ always working within you . . . you work miracles in the world by healing the sick . . . receiving gifts from Christ our Savior, who grants us great mercy.
>
> . . . freely you have received, freely give to us.

We see here an undercurrent of opposition to the practitioners of rational medicine who refused to treat those unable to pay. In such situations the poor found that their only recourse was the unmercenary physician-saint. Many honored such saints, as witnessed by not only the many churches of St. Panteleimon, but most significantly, the richly endowed Russian monastery of St. Panteleimon on the Holy Mountain Athos.

Nevertheless, Christ was seen as the source of their healing powers, whether through medicine or prayers. One of the hymns from the services of the physician-saints Cyrus and John, commemorated on January 31, keeps the divine dimension vividly present: "Having received the gift of miracles from divine grace, O Saints, you work wonders unceasingly, cutting out all our diseases and passions by invisible surgery, O divinely wise Cyrus with glorious John. For you are divine healers."

The mention of "passions," a code-word for sinful attitudes and living, indicates that the healing of the physician-saints was not only of the body. So it is that in the dismissal hymn of the service of St. Panteleimon, no mention is made of bodily healing; the petition is that the saint "intercede with the merciful God that He grant unto our souls forgiveness of sins." In another major hymn of the morning service of St. Panteleimon (the Kontakion), he is implored "by thy prayers heal the diseases of our souls." The spiritual and the physical are always in close proximity, even in the case of the physician-saints, who are repeatedly described as pointing to the interrelatedness of the health of body, soul, and spirit, much as does Lederer's fictional bishop-physician.

HEALING THROUGH LIVING SAINTS

A saint does not necessarily require a medical pedigree in order to have healing powers and to gain fame in the church as a healer. On the contrary, the physician-saints are a minority. Many more healings are claimed as a result of the intercessions of other kinds of saints in the life of the church. In fact, one historian of saints indicates that healing is the chief mark of a saint. But even nonmedically trained saints availed themselves of practices from rational medicine in healing those who came to them.

> Perhaps the commonest manifestation of holiness is the healing power of the saint. He deals with every physical and mental affliction from constipation to leprosy, cancer and gangrene. Usually he works by touch, often accompanied by prayer. Sometimes prayer alone suffices. Sometimes the holy man works his cure at a distance by sending to the patient something which has been in contact with his person. . . . Often the healing offered by the saint is contrasted with that of orthodox doctors. It is instantaneous, while theirs is slow, it is painless while theirs involves much discomfort or the agony of surgery without an anesthetic, and so on. But sometimes there seems to be a tacit demarcation agreement between the holy man and the doctor, who send one another suitable patients.[9]

Thus the holy man and the doctor often treated the same patient and even made referrals to one another. According to another historian of saints and medicine in early Byzantine society, "the holy man becomes one healer among many, prominent in the medical landscape of his area, but not, as a source of medicine or medical advice, wholly different from local physicians."[10]

Many stories from the lives of the saints show the wide range of their relationships with rational medicine. In these sources the saints can be depicted as very antagonistic toward rational medicine, as totally independent of it, and sometimes as quite cooperative. The seventh-century *Life of St. Theodore of Sykeon* describes the practice of a popular saint totally untrained in rational medicine.

Again, if any required medical treatment for certain illnesses, or surgery or purging draught or hot springs, this God-inspired man would prescribe the appropriate remedy to each like an experienced doctor trained in the art. He might recommend one to have recourse to surgery and would always state clearly which doctor he should employ. In other cases he would dissuade those who wished to have an operation or to undergo some other medical treatment, and would recommend rather that they should visit hot springs, and would name the springs they should go to.[11]

But often the "medicine" consisted of such actions as touching the sick person, praying over him or her, sprinkling dust from around the domicile of the saint, or placing on the sick part a cloth that had been in contact with the saint's body.[12] Faith, prayer, rational medicine, magical practices, intuition, and suggestion all seemed to have been mixed together.

Even in their use of dust and touching and instructions to do certain actions, however, the saints took their model from Christ and the early apostolic tradition as recorded in the Gospels and the Book of Acts. For example, in healing a blind man Jesus "spat on the ground and made clay of the spittle and anointed the man's eyes with clay, saying to him, 'Go wash in the pool of Siloam.' . . . So he went and washed and came back seeing" (John 9:6–7). Also, in the New Testament the faithful are described as approaching the apostles for healing: "they even carried out the sick into the streets, and laid them on beds and pallets, that as Peter came by at least his shadow might fall on some of them. The people also gathered from the towns around Jerusalem, bringing the sick and those afflicted with unclean spirits, and they were all healed" (Acts 5:15–16). The use of articles of clothing for healing purposes is not unknown in the New Testament, either: "God did extraordinary miracles by the hands of Paul, so that handkerchiefs or aprons were carried away from his body to the sick, and diseases left them and the evil spirits came out of them" (Acts 18:11–12). Yet the same passage sharply distinguishes this practice from "magic arts," which are strongly rejected (Acts 18:18–19). In consequence, the saint's intercessory activity on the part of the sick was perceived as a continuation of dominical and apostolic traditions.[13]

The most common practice in the stories of the living saints, however, is direct prayer. A sick person is brought to the saint, he prays, and a healing takes place. This procedure clearly continues the tradition of the majority of healings of Christ and the apostles as described in the New Testament. Let one example suffice. According to the editors of his *vita*, St. Nicholas of Sion "flourished in the first half of the sixth century, and like Nicholas of Myra, was active in Lycia; he was abbot of the Monastery of Holy Sion near Myra and was subsequently ordained bishop of Pinara in western Lycia." Among the many healings described in the *Life* is this one:

> One day, [there came] a certain woman from the hamlet of Nikapo who was withered from the unclean spirit, and her husband carried her and brought her to the monastery, and he cast her down at the feet of the holy man. The servant of God prayed to God, and the evil spirit withdrew from her, and she was made whole. And from that very hour she went home on her own feet giving thanks to God and to Holy Sion.[14]

SHRINES OF HEALING SAINTS

The existence of living healing saints is supplemented by the cult of the departed healing saints. They are appealed to in the hymns of their feasts and in some cases at their shrines.

Much attention was given to saints adorned with the healer's reputation, and shrines have been constructed in their honor throughout the church's history. Often such shrines were found in the monasteries where hospitals were also established. While the hospital was the domain of the physician, the shrine was the domain of the saint-healer. But they were not always functionally separate. In most cases, neither the monks nor the physicians nor the patients and their families perceived a sharp line of demarcation between the shrine and the hospital, between what we are calling here spiritual healing and rational medicine.

Ill people would come to the shrine of the healing saint, put down their cot or pallet, and live in the shrine for days or weeks with the expectation that the saint would visit them in the church and heal them, or at least guide them to healing. A vision of the saint in a dream often would be adequate to bring about a healing. Sometimes physicians in the monastery hospital would send a patient to the shrine for the saint's healing intercessions; sometimes the saint in a dream would send a sick person to the hospital.[15]

The tradition of seeking healing at a shrine continues to this day. Many such shrines are to be found in various local Orthodox churches. In Greece, for example, one of the most famous is the Church of the Annunciation of the Virgin Mary, on the Aegean island of Tenos. In 1823, during the first years of the Greek War of Independence, an icon of the Virgin Mary was found during the construction of a church. The icon became the focal point of the shrine, and eventually the shrine became the site of a nationwide annual pilgrimage. Each year thousands make pilgrimage to the shrine, many of whom seek healing from the Virgin. Many have been healed, as is witnessed by great numbers of crutches and votive offerings in the church. These are regularly reported in the nation's press, and archives are maintained of the healings. Accounts of these healings are quite detailed, giving the names and addresses of those healed and the dates of the healings as well as the illness from which they were healed.[16]

In recent years similar shrines have come into existence in the United States; for example, the Shrine of St. Nectarius in Covina, California, the Shrine of the Neomartyr Saints Raphael, Nicholas, and Irene in Astoria, New York, and, perhaps the best known, the Shrine of St. Paraskevi in Greenlawn, New York. In an interview with the priest in charge of the Shrine of St. Paraskevi, I was informed that the shrine, functioning as a "daughter shrine" of the original Shrine of St. Paraskevi at Therapia, outside the walls of Constantinople, Turkey, brings holy water from there annually. According to the pastor, the first cure to take place was the healing of a Jewish woman. Though the majority of pilgrims are Orthodox, many other faiths are also represented in the 3,000–4,000 people who attend during the Feast of St. Paraskevi, annually on July 26. The pastor assured me that many healings have taken place, especially of eye diseases (St. Paraskevi is known as a patron of those who suffer from diseases of the eyes) and of cancer. Nevertheless, he seeks to avoid sensationalism regarding these healings: "we feel that miracles are personal and private."[17]

Most recently, on December 6, 1986, an icon of the Virgin Mary (the Theotokos, or "birth-giver of God") on the iconostasis of a small Albanian Orthodox Church in Chicago began unexpectedly to "weep": fluid began to stream from the eyes of the icon, a canvas painting mounted on a wood panel. The event was interpreted by Archbishop Iakovos of the Greek Orthodox archdiocese as a sign for all persons to "awaken from the sleep of materialism and to nourish themselves spiritually." Within three months of the appearance of the tears 300,000 pilgrims, of all faiths and none, visited the church. As I entered the church proper from the side of the building, I saw a sign which read "Only children and the very ill will be anointed with the tears," giving graphic testimony to the pilgrims' belief that the tears may mediate healing. Several healings have been reported and attributed to the spiritual mediation of "Our Lady of Chicago." The pastor of the church, Father Philip Koufos, has assured me in conversation that he has witnessed several such healings.[18]

POPULAR PIETY AND HYMNS

The veneration of relics of saints and martyrs is also part of the Orthodox tradition. Some of these relics have the reputation of mediating the

cures of diverse illnesses. The conviction is a very old one. St. Gregory of
Nyssa describes the reverence for the relics of martyrs and saints in the
fourth century. One ancient document, for example, describes the discovery of the relics of St. Stephen as having taken place in December of 451.
With the discovery of the Protomartyr's relics "seventy-three people (it is
asserted) were cured of sundry ailments, before the martyr's body was sol-
emnly laid to rest. . . . "[19]

As with St. Paraskevi, who is approached for the healing of eye illnesses,
other saints also have the reputation among the faithful for healing special-
ties. Thus tradition calls upon St. Eleutherius for a safe childbirth; St. Barbara for protection from sudden death; Holy Martyr Boniface and the
Righteous Aglais against drunkenness; the Holy New Martyr Demas of
Smyrna to cure headaches; St. Spyridon the Wonderworker for diseased
ears; St. Antipas of Pergamum for protection of teeth; the Holy Great Martyr Artemius for the healing of hernia and intestinal disorders; St. Blaise of
Sebastea for correction of throat illnesses; St. Gerasimus of Cephalonia, St.
Anastasia, and St. Naum of Ochrid for the curing of mental disorders; St.
Haralambus and St. Marina against plagues. Interestingly enough, both
the Greek and the Slavic traditions have saints who are called upon to
intercede for physicians as well: St. Panteleimon and all the Holy Unmercenaries and St. Agapit the Physician of Kievo-Pechersk.[20]

Appeals to saints for healing are frequent in the worship of the church,
appearing in hundreds of hymns. The most dramatic and specific appeals
are made to those identified as healing saints. For example, one hymn of
the vespers of Sts. Cosmas and Damian mentions the power of the relics of
the saints and their names: it affirms that healing is finally from Christ and
that the objects of healing are spiritual as well as physical diseases.

> Endless is the grace which the saints have received from Christ. There-
> fore, their relics ceaselessly work miracles by this divine strength. Even
> their names, pronounced with faith, heal incurable diseases. By their
> intercessions, O Lord, free us from spiritual and physical ailments, for
> Thou lovest humankind.[21]

St. Anastasia, although not a physician-saint, is known as the *pharma-
kolytreia*, the healer of poisoning. A church bearing her name is described
in a hymn in the morning service of her feast day as a place of healing.
Another hymn from the same service ascribes to her the use of medications for healing the soul, as well as the ability to heal those who have
been poisoned in the body.

They that are in temptations and afflictions hasten to thy temple and receive holy restoration by the divine grace that dwelleth in thee, O Anastasia. For thou dost ever pour forth healing for the world.

By thy sacred potions and medicines, thou, O Anastasia, bringest healing unto our soul and dost cure all suffering from poisoning of the body; for this cause, we acclaim the great grace bestowed on thee.[22]

One of the three chief means of spiritual healing among Orthodox Christians, then, is the appeal to saintly persons to intercede on their behalf for healing at the throne of God. It is not possible, however, to make a clear demarcation between appeals to saints for healing and the liturgical expressions of spiritual healing, as the next chapter demonstrates.

·9·

Spiritual Healing: The Liturgy

In *The Orthodox Church*, Bishop Kallistos Ware begins his discussion of Orthodox worship with a story, taken from the ninth-century *Russian Primary Chronicle*, about the visits of Prince Vladimir's emissaries to various regions in their search for a suitable religion for the people:

> Finally they journeyed to Constantinople, and here at last, as they attended the Divine Liturgy in the great Church of the Holy Wisdom, they discovered what they desired. "We know not whether we were in heaven or on earth, for surely there is no such splendour or beauty anywhere upon the earth. We cannot describe it to you: only this we know, that God dwells there among men, and that their service surpasses the worship of all other places. For we cannot forget that beauty."[1]

The story may or may not be apocryphal, but it points to what is central in Orthodox Christian life: worship. In particular the sacramental life of the Orthodox church is understood to be inseparable from the Orthodox ethos. It is in worship and the sacraments that Orthodox Christians find their identity and their appropriation of the saving work of Jesus Christ in their lives. In a wide range of "divine services"—those centered on the major sacraments and an almost unlimited collection of daily, seasonal, and occasional services and prayers—worshippers attend to the sanctification of the whole of life and focus on the relationship of the faithful with God.

The main focus of the services is spiritual, but not exclusively so; nearly all the services of the church include some mention of healing. The basic library for worship in the Orthodox church, about seventeen volumes, offers rich material for exploring the relationship of the Orthodox Christian faith tradition and issues of health and medicine.[2] This chapter focuses on some of the sacraments, the Supplicatory Service to the Theotokos, and other priestly ministrations, as well as on some popular practices like fasting.

HEALING IN THE SACRAMENTS

Although physical and bodily health is not central to the concerns of the sacraments, neither is it completely absent. The sacraments are experiences of the life of God's kingdom and a manifestation of it in this world, and the dimensions of healing are part of the life of the kingdom as well.[3] Three sacraments—baptism, the Divine Liturgy (the Eucharist), and holy confession—contain expressions of Orthodoxy's concern for well-being and the healing of illness.

The Sacrament of Baptism. The baptismal sacrament begins with a service known as the Making of a Catechumen (or the Instruction), which originated in the early church for the reception of the catechumens. The catechumens had been receiving instruction prior to their baptism and were now ready to be included in the church in full membership. Baptism served to accomplish this (and other things as well).

The service includes exorcisms and a dialogue in which sin, evil, and the devil are rejected. This dialogue is followed by the acceptance of Christ. In one of the exorcisms Jesus Christ is appealed to as the one "who heals every sickness and every infirmity."[4] In the baptismal service proper, the candidate is immersed in water made holy through the "Prayer of the Blessing of the Baptismal Waters." Over the baptismal water the priest prays, "Make it a fountain, a gift of sanctification, a loosing of sins, able to protect from sicknesses."[5]

Clearly, the central focus of the baptismal service is the incorporation of the candidate into the body of the church, not the healing of physical illnesses. But even in this rite, the perspective of healing and health is present and is included in this sacramental action. So it is with other sacraments of the church.

The Sacrament of the Eucharist. The Divine Liturgy of St. John Chrysostom, the central service of worship in the Orthodox church (the Eucharist), also refers to healing only tangentially. The focus is rather on life in the kingdom and the spiritual unity of the believer in the church with Christ and his people. Nevertheless, certain petitions and other portions of the service's text refer specifically to well-being, health, illness, and healing. Because the Divine Liturgy is so central to Orthodox church life, it is worthwhile to list some of these references.[6]

The text of the Divine Liturgy of St. John Chrysostom includes petitions for the sick and the suffering and for health and well-being. Thus, we hear in the litany at the beginning of the service: "For travelers by land, sea and air, for the sick, the suffering, the captives, and for their salvation, let us pray to the Lord." Following the consecration, the priest also specifically indicates that the Eucharist is offered for the sick and the suffering, among others. "Remember, Lord," he prays, "the travelers, the sick, the suffering, and the captives, granting them protection and salvation." In the prayer of thanksgiving following the consecration of the gifts in the Divine Liturgy of St. Basil, a similar request is made: "Remember, Lord, the people present here . . . nourish the babes, instruct the youth, console the elderly; comfort the feeble minded. . . . Free those who are bothered by unclean spirits . . . heal the sick."[7]

In anticipation of receiving the Eucharist, at the "Prayer of the Bowing of the Head," a prayer for healing is offered. Perhaps more clearly and forcefully than at any other place in the Divine Liturgy of St. John Chrysostom, this prayer speaks to the need for healing in a fully Christ-centered way: "Therefore, Master, guide the course of our life for our benefit according to the need of each of us. Sail with those who sail; travel with those who travel; and heal the sick, Physician of our souls and bodies." Following the Divine Liturgy, those who have participated in Holy Communion may repeat the several prayers of thanksgiving. Within them we find these words: "O loving Master, who died and rose for our sake, and granted to us these awesome and life-giving mysteries for the well-being and sanctification of our souls and bodies, let these gifts be for a healing of my own soul and body, the averting of every evil. . . . "[8]

From the time of the earliest Fathers and teachers of the church, Holy Communion has been termed a *pharmakon*, or medicine. The term was used by Serapion, the fourth-century bishop of Thmuis in Egypt, in reference to Holy Communion as a "medicine of life," and it was described as a "medicine of immortality" by Ignatius in his *Letter to the Ephesians*.[9]

The Sacrament of Repentance. The sacrament least likely to be associated with physical healing is the sacrament of repentance, or confession, because its main concern is forgiveness of sins and spiritual regeneration. The order of service for the sacrament of repentance is quite fluid, even today; it varies from service book to service book. None of the numerous prayers for forgiveness, however, addresses the issue of physical illness. In some cases, the Greek word *astheneia*, often translated as "sickness" or "illness," is used in the prayers, but the context makes clear that "human weakness" is meant, not specific physical or emotional illness.

In this metaphorical sense of healing, though, the sacrament sometimes is paralleled with the curing of physical illnesses. No less an authority than the Sixth Ecumenical Council of 692 makes such a parallel between the work of the father-confessor and the physician of bodily ills.

It is incumbent upon those who have received from God the power to bind and to loose, to consider the quality of the sin and the readiness of the sinner for conversion, and to apply medicine suitable for the disease, lest if he is injudicious in each of these respects he should fail in regard to the healing of the sick man. For the disease of sin is not simple but various and multiform, and it germinates many mischievous offshoots, from which much evil is diffused, and it proceeds further until it is checked by the power of the physician. Therefore he who professes the science of spiritual medicine first of all should consider the disposition of him who has sinned, and to see whether he tends to health or, on the contrary, provokes his disease by his own behavior, and to look how he can care for his manner of life during the interval. And if he does not resist the physician, and if the ulcer of the soul is increased by application of the imposed medicaments, then let him mete out mercy on him.[10]

This aspect of healing is captured well by author and lecturer Constantine Cavarnos, who describes the work of the father-confessor as "spiritual diagnosis, spiritual mid-wifery, spiritual surgery, and spiritual therapy."[11]

But others have seen and emphasized the actual connection between spiritual illness and physical distress. Given the possible relationships between sin and sickness discussed above, it is fully understandable that the therapeutic model would appeal to those dealing with the sacrament of holy confession and the connection of sin to physical illness, though one must be very careful not to do this in a mechanical and arbitrary way. To affirm the "psychosomatic connection" between some instances of sinful living and physical illness is not to say that every physical illness is directly caused by a specific sin. Nevertheless, it was Chrysostom who taught— perhaps with some rhetorical exaggeration—that "most of our diseases arise from sins of the soul. For if the sum of all, death itself, hath its root and foundation from sin, much more the majority of our diseases also: since our very capability of suffering did itself originate there."[12]

Thus even a sacramental practice that is far removed from healing practices as normally understood finds itself used for healing purposes.

ANOINTING AND THE SUPPLICATORY SERVICE

The life of the Orthodox church is rich with services and liturgical practices that bear directly or indirectly on care for the sick. Within Orthodoxy itself, some practices are more dominant among the Greek and Antiochian traditions, and others are more widespread among the churches of the Slavic Orthodox tradition. The anointing with oil from vigil lamps is part of the Slavic tradition, while the Service of the Small Paraklesis to the Most Holy Theotokos is used in Greek and Antiochian churches.

A popularly written booklet regarding home practices of the faith, coming from a traditional Russian Orthodox source, provides a perspective on the use of oil in this religious tradition. "The anointing with oil takes place in the Mysteries of Baptism and Holy Unction and at the All-night Vigil Service on the eves of important feasts." Its connection with healing follows:

> Oil symbolizes God's mercy and when used in anointing it is a visible embodiment of the grace of healing. Christians, therefore, often keep small bottles of holy oil in their icon corner and anoint themselves and others of their family with the sign of the Cross in Holy Oil. This anointing is usually done on the individual's forehead.[13]

Most prized is oil from vigil lamps in shrines, special churches, or other places where saints are buried, or from vigil lamps burning before miraculous icons. In the Slavic tradition this oil is popularly used much as the oils of the sacrament of holy unction are used. Though this tradition is not widespread among the Greek-speaking Orthodox, it does have some currency.

In contrast, wide use is made in the Greek and Antiochian Orthodox traditions of a service directed to the Theotokos—to Mary, the "birth-giver of God." The Supplicatory Service (Greek, *Paraklesis*) is most frequently conducted in the church building or in homes. The Theotokos, the first and chief of all the saints in the Orthodox tradition, is perceived as a protectress. One of the hymns of the service, in a metric translation, chants as follows: "I have sought refuge in you; / O Mother of the Word and ever-Virgin, / From all distresses and dangers deliver me."[14]

In addition to numerous general appeals for deliverance from dangers, relief from grief, sorrow, temptations, and so on, the hymns offer many specific petitions for healing from sickness; seven such hymns appear in the service which are unique to it.[15] For example, one hymn, while including the consistent teaching of Orthodox Christianity that God is the real healer of illness, makes this affirmation together with an appeal to the Theotokos for intercession for healing.

> I lie now on a bed of infirmities,
> And there is no healing at all for my body
> Except for you,
> Who has brought forth our Savior,
> God, the healer of all our infirmities;

Of your goodness, I pray to you,
From corruption of sicknesses raise me.[16]

Another hymn captures in a few lines of pathos the psychological effects of
illness on the human spirit and relates it to the theme of wholeness:

Oppressed I am, O Virgin;
In a place of sickness,
I have been humbled; I ask you: bring remedy,
Transform my illness, my sickness,
Into wholesomeness.[17]

Another hymn in the service expresses the psychosomatic relation of illness and sin. It is, as was pointed out above, improper to relate every
illness to a specific sin. Yet certainly in some situations sins are directly
related to particular illnesses and diseases of both the psyche and the
body. Nowhere is this truth more clearly expressed in Orthodox liturgical
practice than in this hymn from the Supplicatory Service:

From the great multitude of my sins,
Ill am I in body,
Ill am I also in my soul;
I am fleeing to you,
The one who is all-blessed,
The hope of the hopeless,
Please come, bring help to me.[18]

Here we speak of such sins as gluttony, which may lead to internal organ
debilitation and early death; abuse of alcohol, which may cause cirrhosis of
the liver; sexual promiscuity, which leads to venereal and other diseases;
and jealousy, the lack of forgiveness for wrongs suffered, or an unrelieved
spirit of vengeance, which may lead to personality disorders. Both experience and the wholistic approach to life embodied in the Orthodox Christian tradition force acknowledgment of this aspect of sin and health.

FASTING AND HEALTH

The Orthodox church observes frequent fast periods. Often apparent
conflicts may arise concerning medications and fasting practices. It is important to note that the meaning of *fasting* as complete avoidance of all
food (other than water) for a specific period of time had largely been abandoned in the Orthodox church; the exception is fasting from midnight to

the reception of Holy Communion. In the early church, fasting for longer periods meant not eating anything from sunup to sundown, but such fasting is practiced in the Orthodox world today only in monasteries.

Nevertheless, fasting periods are scattered throughout the church calendar and are honored by many Orthodox. During these, abstinence from certain foods is observed. The four long-term fasts are these: (1) the Great Lent before Easter, including Palm Sunday and Holy Week, a period of forty-seven days; (2) the Christmas fast, of forty days; (3) the Fast of the Holy Apostles, varying in length, but approximately seven to ten days; and (4) the two-week fast preceding the Feast of the Dormition of the Theotokos, celebrated annually on August 15. The shorter fasts may also be categorized: (1) Wednesdays and Fridays of nearly all weeks of the year; (2) the fast day before the Feast of the Epiphany (January 5); (3) the fast day of the Feast of the Holy Cross (September 14); and (4) fasts relating to particular saints' days, such as the Beheading of St. John the Baptist, on August 29.[19]

The fasts vary in severity depending on the foods being abstained from. Very roughly, from the least strict to the most strict, the list is as follows: meat of all kinds; milk, cheese, other dairy products, and eggs; fish; shellfish; oil; wine; and "dry eating," that is, bread, vegetables, and dried fruits like raisins, dates, and nuts, as well as fresh fruits. These levels of strictness are often related to the nature of the fast. For example, the weekly fasts on Wednesdays and Fridays are much less severe than those of the Holy Cross or Great Lent.[20]

The connection of these fast periods with issues of health is twofold. On the one hand, though all Orthodox Christians are urged to fast, it is not permitted for one who is ill to fast so as to cause physical harm to himself or herself. Thus a late-fourth-century canon, endorsed by an Ecumenical Council and therefore having full validity in the Orthodox church, orders all Christians to fast during the Great Lent, as well as on Wednesdays and Fridays, unless "prevented from doing so by reason of bodily illness." Exceptions are also made in the canonical tradition for pregnant women and those giving birth during fast periods, the very young, and the infirm elderly. Preachers and commentators frequently caution, however, that minor or imagined illnesses ought not be used as an excuse for avoiding fasting.[21] They maintain, rather, that fasting for religious and spiritual reasons helps preserve bodily health. In a full-length study on the institution of fasting in the Orthodox church, Chrestos M. Enisleides devotes the epilogue to the positive effects of fasting on health, although he is fully aware that fasting is mainly for spiritual purposes, for self-discipline and self-control.[22]

OTHER PRIESTLY MINISTRATIONS FOR HEALTH

Other elements in the liturgical tradition of the Orthodox church also address illness and sickness.

Included in the various prayer books used by the Orthodox clergy are several prayers for the sick. One prayer used rather widely is directed to God the Father as "the healer of our souls and bodies":

> O Lord Almighty, the Healer of our souls and bodies, You who put down and raise up, Who chastise and heal also; do You now, in Your great mercy, visit our brother (sister) (Name), who is sick. Stretch forth Your hand that is full of healing and health, and get him (her) up from his (her) bed, and cure him (her) of his (her) illness. Put away from him (her) the spirit of disease and of every malady, pain and fever to which he (she) is bound; and if he (she) has sins and transgressions, grant to him (her) remission and forgiveness, in that You love humankind; yea, Lord my God, pity Your creation, through the compassions of Your Only-Begotten Son, together with Your All-Holy, Good and Life-creating Spirit, with Whom You are blessed, both now and ever, and to the ages of ages. Amen.[23]

The highlights of this prayer are clear: God is the healer; sickness is an evil to be healed; some connection between it and sin is acknowledged; God is compassionate regarding our suffering; and he is philanthropically disposed toward us, so that we may appeal to him for healing.

A practice becoming increasingly familiar in parish life is the repetition of the prayer "Lord Jesus Christ, Son of God, have mercy on me." Known as the "Jesus Prayer," it comes out of the Hesychast spiritual tradition of Orthodox monasticism, which is illustrated and embodied in *The Philokalia*. In monastic practice, the goal is to repeat the prayer until it "prays itself" in the heart, so fulfilling the command to "pray constantly" (*adialeiptos*, that is, "without interruption," "unceasingly"). The practice is based on St. Paul's instruction as recorded in 1 Thessalonians 5:17.

Since the end of the Second World War, there has developed in Orthodox Christianity a strong movement of "returning to the traditions of the Fathers," a reaction to the "Westernization" that took place in Orthodoxy as a result of the influence of Peter the Great, tsar of Russia. Return to earlier traditional patterns of iconography, music, architecture, and spiritual life also provoked an interest in monasticism and in monastic prayer patterns like the Jesus Prayer. As the practice of the Jesus Prayer has become known in parish life, priests are beginning to recommend it to laypeople to strengthen their personal spiritual lives and to help them in times of stress like illness, hospitalization, and surgery.

Other practices are used in the liturgical sphere to aid healing. Exorcisms, prayers for the expulsion of evil spirits and influences, are commonly found in the service books and are available to the clergy when the need is felt. Priests have recounted to me dramatic and striking instances when the Service of Exorcism was read for mentally ill persons with beneficial effect during the Service of the Proskomide, the service of preparation before the Divine Liturgy.[24] I was once asked to remove my vestments after the Divine Liturgy and to place them upon the head and shoulders of a sick person who had been brought to the church. After I did so three times, the woman returned to normal behavior and life in the parish for about three years; later some of her symptoms returned. We then repeated the procedure, and the woman again experienced improvement in her condition. Prayers are also offered for those who perceive themselves as suffering from the influence of the "evil eye." (In the area of the Eastern Mediterranean, it is widely believed that certain persons have the ability to bring sickness or harm to others simply by looking upon them with evil intent.)[25] Concern for the ill is also expressed in the short booklets containing prayers and spiritual guidance that are issued by individual priests and by Orthodox clergy brotherhoods and associations.[26]

Finally, the popular Service for the Blessing of the Waters is also often used for therapeutic purposes. Water is blessed during the Epiphany observance of the baptism of Christ; water is sanctified at the beginning of the baptismal service for Christians; water is added to the chalice for Holy Communion. In addition, water is blessed and sprinkled upon all manner of objects and human conditions. Some of the hymns and prayers of the water-blessing service reflect the themes of the hymns considered above in Chapter 8. The following hymn addresses the Virgin Mary:

> From every sickness and infirmity, deliver us, who have recourse to you and your holy Protection.
>
> Your Temple, O Theotokos, was shown forth as remedy of ills without pay—the consolation of our wounded souls.
>
> From every ban under which they labor deliver your servants; from every ailment of body and spirit, O you most Holy.[27]

Following the reading of the Gospel passage on the healing at the pool of Bethesda (John 5:1–4), however, the theme of the healing power of blessed water comes to the fore. The litany asks "that this water may be to the healing of souls and bodies, and to the banishment of every hostile power." The prayer immediately following appeals to Christ who came into the world, "in the similitude of a servant, scorning not our image but giving true health to the body and saying, 'Lo! You are healed, sin no more.'" Reference is made in the prayer to the healing of the blind man at the pool of Siloam (John 9:1–12), which leads to an impassioned plea for healing: "Yea, we beseech You visit our weaknesses, O Good One, and heal our infirmities both of spirit and the body through Your mercy." The prayer ends with the ascription "For You are the Fountain of healing, O Christ our God, and to You we send up glory."[28]

The services of the Orthodox church are thus replete with a sense of the potential for spiritual healing. Whether appealing directly to Christ, or indirectly through the saints, they look to God as a ready source of healing. It is Christ, finally, who is seen as the true "Physician of our souls and bodies." Perhaps this hymn from the early part of the Service for the Blessing of the Waters adequately expresses the gist of the concern for spiritual healing in the liturgical life and practice of the Orthodox church:

> O Christ, the Fountain, Who did sprinkle the waters of healing in the all-holy Temple of the Virgin, You, today, through the sprinkling of blessing did expel the maladies of those who are sick, O You Physician of our souls and bodies.[29]

· 10 ·

Spiritual Healing: Holy Unction

The Orthodox Christian tradition embraces all dimensions of our existence within the saving, redeeming, sanctifying work of Christ and the church. Clearly, exorcisms, the efforts of rational medicine, the healings of the saints, and the concern for the sick shown in liturgical life (and in the sacrament of healing specifically) indicate that the Orthodox church is concerned with the health and well-being of the sick and suffering. It would be a serious mistake, on the one hand, to interpret these efforts as mere "alternative therapies" which could be dispensed with now that scientific medicine is so advanced. Nor would it be correct, on the other hand, to "spiritualize" them into mere paradigms of the kingdom, without application to the empirical human condition.[1] We may not discount what the sacraments mean for the concrete bodily, spiritual, psychological, and communal aspects of human life. This would be a distortion and denial of the incarnational dimension of Christianity.

Thus the sacrament of healing must be seen in its kingdom context but also in its concreteness and interrelatedness with the experienced reality of human illness—spiritual, psychological, and physical. Orthodox Christianity cares so much about sickness, in all of its dimensions, that it has a sacrament dedicated to healing. The sacrament of healing (known also as the sacrament of prayer oil, unction, or holy oil) has in the Orthodox tradition continuously retained its healing character, in contradistinction to other Christian traditions which historically have either turned it into a rite for the dead or rejected it completely.

THE SACRAMENT OF HEALING IN HISTORY

Students of the development of the liturgies of Holy Communion describe a process, during the first four centuries of the Christian church, in which many liturgical structures and practices little by little coalesced into just a handful of Divine Liturgies used in church worship. In the Eastern

99

Orthodox church, only four remain in practice: the liturgies of St. John Chrysostom, St. Basil, and St. James (Iakovos) and the Liturgy of the Presanctified Gifts.

Something similar happened with the sacrament of healing in the Eastern Christian tradition, except that the process remained fluid much longer and the sacrament retained its essential form much longer. Evidence suggests that certain external circumstances, around the tenth and eleventh centuries, caused the church in several steps to expand the rite and to give it a much more impressive and dramatic form.

The use of oil for healing purposes has a long tradition. The Greeks and Romans used it thus, as did the Jews; the anointing of the sick is mentioned in the Talmud.[2]

The Gospels make several references to the use of oil and to anointing, but in only one instance is an anointing with oil explicitly related to healing: in Mark 6:13 the Twelve on their missionary journey "cast out many demons, and anointed with oil many that were sick and healed them." The Good Samaritan's pouring of oil on the wounds of the thieves' victim seems to have this purpose as well (Luke 10:30–37).

The early Christian tradition accepted the passage in James 5:14 as the authoritative foundation for the sacrament of healing.

> Is any among you sick? Let him call for the elders [Greek, *tous presbyterous*] of the church, and let them pray over him, anointing him with oil in the name of the Lord; and the prayer of faith will save the sick man, and the Lord will raise him up; and if he has committed sins, he will be forgiven.

At least four elements are part of the action described here. First, this is not a casual or private anointing. In the case of illness, a sick person is instructed to call for officials of the church. It is generally accepted that we are already talking about clergy, those persons set aside and ordained as assistants to the local bishop. The anointing is an action of the church. Second, the anointing of a sick person's body with oil is a physical act, a familiar therapeutic tradition of that time and age. Third, nevertheless, the anointing is not merely a simple medical procedure: it is associated with prayer, as is the case with every other sacramental action. It combines intimately the material and spiritual elements to form a single sacramental act. And fourth, it is related to the forgiveness of sins, indicating not only the connection between sickness and sin but also the spiritual dimensions of this act of healing.

Some scholars believe it probable that the earliest blessing over oil is found in the Coptic fragment of the *Didache* (c. 150) and that in all likelihood this oil was used for healing purposes.[3] Hippolytus, in his *Apostolic Tradition* (c. 215), includes a reference to the blessing of oil and its use for purposes of health: in a prayer for the blessing of oil, a petition to God is made to "sanctify this oil so that it may give strength to all that taste of it and health to all that use it."[4]

There is evidence in the early Byzantine Empire that oil was blessed for the spiritual healing of physical ailments. Origen (185–254?) closely connects the penitential and healing aspects of the sacrament,[5] and the fourth-century Aphaates the Syrian (c. 350) indicates that oil was blessed for spiritual healing purposes.[6]

An important document regarding the history of the sacrament of healing in the early church is a letter of Innocent I of Rome (416), because it indicates both the earlier practice of anointing by priests (presbyters) and a new practice of allowing the laity to anoint the sick with unction. In a letter to Decentius on the topic of the administration of the sacrament, Innocent writes that "the faithful who are sick can be anointed with the holy oil of unction, which has been prepared by the bishop and which not only priests but all Christians may use for anointing, when their own needs or those of their family demand."[7]

From the fourth-century *Sacramentary of Serapion*, it is clear that the blessing of the oil did not then take place in a separate, distinct, and fully formed service but at some place in the liturgy of the Eucharist. Serapion's prayer becomes the source for the prayer of the consecration of the oil in the subsequent history of the Eastern Orthodox tradition. In part, it reads

> we pray Thee to send down from the heavens of thy Only-begotten a curative power upon this oil, in order that to those who are anointed [with it] . . . it may become a means of removing "every disease and every sickness," of warding off every demon, of putting to flight every unclean spirit, of keeping at a distance every evil spirit, of banishing all fever, all chill, and all weariness; a means of grace and goodness and the remission of sins; a medicament of life and salvation, unto health and soundness of soul and body and spirit, unto perfect well-being.[8]

There was much flexibility in the administration of the sacrament both in the West and in the East. In the West the sacrament was eventually restricted to use with the dying, a practice changed only in recent years by the decrees of the Roman Catholic Second Vatican Council. The practice in the East continued the blessing and administration of the healing sacrament within the eucharistic celebration for the purpose of healing. In the *Sacramentary of Serapion* is also the beginning of the tradition of two distinct phases of the liturgy of the sacrament of healing: the blessing of the oil and the prayer at the anointing itself. The oldest manuscript traditions of the East locate these prayers within the text of the Divine Liturgy. In the middle Byzantine period, from the ninth through the twelfth centuries, the manuscript tradition continued to indicate the same practice, though the prayers are not always in the same place in the Divine Liturgy.

With the beginning of the late Byzantine period, two important developments take place concurrently that are of interest both to medical practitioners and to concerned Orthodox Christians. On the one hand, after nearly a thousand years of involvement, the church's direct supervision and financing of Byzantium's hospitals came to an end. The medical guilds with imperial support assumed control of the hospitals in the twelfth century, and doctors gradually came to dominate hospital administrations.[9] Thus the church was left without access to the healing of the sick through institutions of rational medicine.

It should not surprise us that the church sought some way of responding to this exclusion from the healing process in the society of that day. In the subsequent century tendencies to enhance the liturgical form of the sacrament of healing led to its separation from the context of the Divine Liturgy and to the formation of a service complete in itself. It is possible to trace the development of this service through the thirteenth, fourteenth, and fifteenth centuries and to show how the present-day pattern of seven Epistle and seven Gospel readings and seven prayers emerged.[10] With the introduction of printed service books the text of the service became more or less fixed.

Nicephorus, patriarch of Constantinople from 1260 to 1261, wrote that his predecessor, Patriarch Arsenius Autoreianus (1255–60), had ordered officially that the sacrament of holy unction be conducted by seven priests, defining also seven prayers to be said during the service. He had also increased the number of biblical readings from two to seven. Some scholars believe that this same Arsenius wrote a canon of hymns especially for the service of prayer oil. Among the last Byzantine hierarchs to contribute to the formation of the sacrament was Symeon, archbishop of Thessalonica (1410–29). A prolific author of both doctrinal and liturgical works, he seems to have contributed prayers for the forgiveness of sins prior to the anointing with the oils during the sacrament of unction.[11]

It appears that the service continued its development even after the fall of Constantinople with the increase of the Scripture readings from seven to fourteen. A late addition to the service is the final reading of a prayer of forgiveness as the metal-bound Gospel book is held open with the pages facing down, over the heads of those for whom the sacrament is being conducted. It would appear, then, that the church itself enhanced and strengthened this service precisely when it lost control of the hospitals, thus expressing its continued commitment to a healing ministry.

THE PRAYERS OF CONSECRATION AND ANOINTING

Orthodox Christians in particular will be interested in the development of the service of holy unction, but it also impinges on the relationship of medical professionals to the healing ministry of the clergy. Over the years, the present rite of the sacrament of healing has drawn upon many of the pre-existing services of the Orthodox church: vespers, orthros (the morning service), the eucharistic liturgy. It has borrowed general hymnology related to Christ as healer and to healing saints and provoked the creation of a hymnological canon; it includes blessings; it has incorporated choice Epistle and Gospel passages; and it brings together various prayers for healing in general, for forgiveness of sins, and for anointing. Several of the elements of the service in use today have significance for our study.[12]

The prayer of consecration is short, beginning with an appeal to the mercies of God, healer of the brokenness of human life. After the invocation that God sanctify the oil so that it might free those anointed with it from the illnesses of the soul and the body and from all kinds of evil, the purpose is articulated—that God's name be praised and glorified. Thus the expected healing is "located" within the reign of God.

> O Lord, in Your mercies and compassion, heal the brokenness of our souls and bodies; do You, the same Master, sanctify this oil, that it may be effectual for those who shall be anointed with it, for healing, and for relief from every passion, every defilement of the flesh and of the spirit, and of every evil; and that through it may be glorified Your most holy name, of the Father, and of the Son, and of the Holy Spirit, now and ever, and to the ages of ages. Amen.[13]

The text makes clear the main purpose of this sacrament as distinguished from other sacraments: the healing of body and spirit, and through the healing, the glorification of God. Twice the wholistic dimension of the sacrament is emphasized, and the order is reversed at each mention (souls-bodies/flesh-spirit). "Passion" is undefined; no doubt it is a comprehensive reference to both sin and suffering. While the use of the word "defilement" (Greek, *molysmos*) places much greater emphasis on sin as a dimension of illness, the phrase "every evil" seems to catch up into a single concept all the dimensions of concern.

It is interesting to juxtapose the prayer of anointing with the prayer of consecration. The priest is instructed to take a cotton-tipped wand and to "anoint the sick person, in cross-form; on the brow, the nostrils, the cheeks, the lips, the breast, and on both sides of the hands, repeating the while this prayer":

> O holy Father, Physician of souls and bodies, Who sent your Only-begotten Son, our Lord Jesus Christ, Who heals every infirmity and delivers from death: Heal also, your servant (name) from the ills of body and soul which hinder him/her, and quicken him/her by the grace of Your Christ; through the prayers of our most holy Lady, the Birth-giver of God and ever-virgin Mary; through the intercession of [here the angels, the holy cross, John the Baptist, the apostles, the martyrs, the holy Fathers, the holy unmercenaries, Joachim and Anna, and "all the Saints" are named]. For You are the fountain of healing, O our God, and to You do we ascribe glory, together with Your Only-begotten Son, and Your Spirit, one in essence, now and ever, and unto ages of ages. Amen.[14]

Here, too, the purpose of the anointing is absolutely clear: the healing of body and soul. This certainly includes forgiveness of sins, but it is impossible to argue from this text that the main purpose is something other than healing, with the evidence strongly pointing to healing of disease. In its own way the prayer of anointing reaffirms the wholistic character of the Orthodox church's concern for health. It is always perceived to be within the total range of the church's experience, never an isolated phenomenon.

THE SCRIPTURE READINGS AND THE PRAYERS

In its present form, the heart of the service consists of a set pattern of seven segments, each of which contains an Epistle reading (from the letters of St. Paul or others in the New Testament), the Gospel reading, and a prayer based more or less on the preceding scriptural passages.

The selection of the Scripture readings for this sacrament is impressive. The readings touch on a range of topics: the institution of the sacrament in the Epistle of James, compassion for the suffering, repentance for sins, healing as a gift, the use of oil for healing, and instances of healing by

Christ. Thus those in attendance hear at the beginning "is any among you sick, let him call the presbyters," the foundation verse for the church's special prayer for those who are ill (James 5:10–17). The story of the Good Samaritan (Luke 10:25–38) indicates to the worshipper the truth that we are responsible for the care of our afflicted neighbor, as an expression of Christian love.

In Romans 15:1–8, the worshipper hears the passage "We that are strong ought to bear the infirmities of the weak and not please ourselves." Also heard is the famous passage on love from 1 Corinthians (12:27–13:8), which also speaks of "gifts of healing." Love and philanthropy are emphasized here. In this context of healing, admonitions concerning sin and moral purity are also communicated. Those in attendance are told "we are the temple of the living God" (2 Corinthians 6:16), intimating the connection of sin with sickness and moral purity with health. The Gospel passage describing the healing of St. Peter's mother-in-law (Matthew 8:14–17) is among several healings included in the readings.

As an encouragement, St. Paul's "deliverance from affliction" is presented to the worshippers, showing the availability of God's mercy to deliver us from concrete situations of physical distress. Here, too, reference is made to intercessory prayer (2 Corinthians 1:8–11). Another passage describes the healing of the daughter of the Canaanite woman (Matthew 15:21–28), and the emphasis of the passage is on her subjective faith: " 'O woman, great is your faith! Be it done for you as you desire.' And her daughter was healed instantly." The last Epistle reading (1 Thessalonians 5:14–23) includes the well-known wholistic blessing of the Apostle Paul: "May the God of peace himself sanctify you wholly; and may your spirit and soul and body be kept sound and blameless at the coming of our Lord Jesus Christ." This passage may be the perfect summary statement of the church's approach to healing. The merciful concern for those in need closes the readings through the passage of the call of St. Matthew and Jesus' retort to his enemies' charge that he was consorting with sinners. The medical analogy to spiritual illness is significantly placed at the end of the readings: "Those who are well have no need of a physician, but those who are sick. Go and learn what this means, 'I desire mercy, and not sacrifice.' For I came not to call the righteous, but sinners" (Matthew 9:9–13).

In summary, these biblical passages are remarkable for their references to the "kingdom context" of healing, to both spiritual healing and rational medicine, to the relation of sin and sickness, to the need for forgiveness of sins, to physical and spiritual healing, to compassion and love for those who suffer, to the need for faith on the part of those who are sick, to the power of God to heal, to the gift of healing in the church, to intercessory prayer for healing, and not least, the use of oil for healing and the existence of a sacrament in the church for healing.

Similarly, the wholistic dimension of the Orthodox approach to health and illness is amply expressed in the seven prayers accompanying the Scripture readings. The prayers begin with an emphasis on the spiritual and the sacramental aspects of the sacrament (the first four mention the sanctification of the oil) and forgiveness of sin. The third and fourth prayers deal almost exclusively with physical healing. The fifth mentions both spiritual and physical healing, and the final two focus on forgiveness of sins in their petitions, while referring to God's healing powers in their ascriptions to him.

THE SACRAMENT OF HEALING IN PASTORAL PRACTICE

A popular book on lay practice of the faith emphasizes spiritual preparation of the family before the service of unction on Holy Wednesday (when it is practiced in the Greek tradition).[15] Conducting the sacrament in the home is universal to all Orthodox, but not extremely common. Sometimes the service is conducted for one who is ill. Many times, however, it is conducted as a general service of blessing—as an act, one might say, of "preventive spiritual medicine." Concerning the use of the sacrament in the former case, an author in the Slavic Orthodox tradition observes,

> The priest should be called during illnesses so that he may pray for the infirm, offer spiritual advice and bring the mysteries of Holy Confession, Holy Communion and Holy Unction. The idea that a priest should be called only when someone is in danger of death is not an Orthodox idea. . . . The priest does not come to prepare a person for the grave but he comes to bring spiritual life. Holy Unction is a service for the spiritual and physical health of an individual."[16]

When clergy of the Greek Orthodox Archdiocese were solicited for comments about the sacrament during the preparation for this book, many responded with a high appreciation of its value in their ministries. One commented that "very, very often both Greek and American-born parishioners are comforted by it and responsive to it." Another noted that "unction provides to sick persons God's grace in a special manner" and that it is "effective, meaningful." One priest remarked that "at home it often provides an opportunity for the whole family to pray for the sick person." Another priest told of the spiritual healing through the sacrament of a young woman who believed she was possessed. A bishop wrote: "Holy

Unction and Holy Confession are important tools in the healing ministry of the Holy Orthodox Church. They help me in my ministry on behalf of the 'Healer of our souls and bodies' a great deal. I wish we would make more use of them as we tend to the health, both physical and spiritual, of the flock of Christ in today's world."

Some priests reserve its use for "very serious illness," while others are quite liberal with it. Thus one priest reported, "I encourage people to be anointed at any time they feel the need or the desire, not only at times of great sickness." Other priests try to extend the impact and spiritual benefit of the service by suggesting devotional practices connected with the anointing; one priest wrote, "I suggest to our people that they read and offer prayerfully several of the unction prayers on an ongoing basis for ensuing weeks."

Several priests commented upon the negative attitudes they experienced in hospital settings, especially when they tried to conduct the whole service at the bedside: they cited "too many distractions, sometimes complete disregard by the medical staff, along with the insensitivity of medical personnel who often feel we are interfering with their patients." Most priests understand how the medical staff feels, and consequently they do not conduct the whole hour-long service in the hospital room. General practice seems to be the reading of a few prayers, one of which is the "Prayer of Anointing," and the anointing of the patient. However, there is no uniformity of practice. Thus the widest use of the sacrament of unction seems to be in the hospital, where the whole service is hardly ever conducted. Rather, the option of using holy oil which has been previously consecrated and reserved for later use is perceived as the only one open to priests in the hospital setting.

THE NEED FOR NEW UNCTION PRACTICES

The remarkable history of this sacrament, its vitality, and the beautiful architecture of its order of service make it one of the most important liturgical and spiritual embodiments of the Orthodox tradition of spiritual healing. But the sacrament witnesses as well to the coexistence of the various traditions of healing within the consciousness and practice of the Orthodox Christian tradition.

Perhaps a careful study of the theology and development of the sacrament of holy unction would move the church's contemporary practice closer to the early form of the sacrament, especially in its connection with the Eucharist. A few priests today are setting an example for conducting the sacrament of healing authentically in the hectic twentieth century. They have the faithful who are about to enter the hospital prepare properly for Holy Communion, attend the Divine Liturgy, receive the Eucharist, and then, either within or after the liturgy (the former is, of course, historically and liturgically more correct), be anointed with the oils of healing, supported by the prayers of the congregation.

In addition, because emergencies sometimes prevent the observance of this procedure, a brief service of anointing may be needed at the hospital bedside. This service could use reserve sacramental unction and have some elements of the contemporary sacramental service: hymns, Scripture, prayers, and the ancient prayer of anointing. If possible, the family members would be in attendance.

Of course, although the healing purpose of the sacrament should not be ignored or relativized, neither should the larger perspective of the sacramental life be forgotten. Every sacrament, including the healing of prayer oil, points to growth in the image and likeness of God, to the acquisition of the Holy Spirit, and to the incorporation of the Body of Christ, his people, into the kingdom of God.

Part IV
PASSAGES AND ETHICS

· 11 ·

Passages: Beginnings

As a society we have recently gained a new awareness of the importance of "passages" in the lives of persons. This sensitivity is especially valuable to those concerned with the health and well-being of others.

What have been the attitudes of the Orthodox church toward the idea of passages in general? How has the church dealt with particular passages— birth, incorporation into the life of the faith community, youth, marriage, family life, maturation, dying, and death? These questions direct the thrust of this final section, which concludes with a treatment of bioethical issues from an Orthodox perspective.

In all these discussions two dimensions of human development are present. On the one hand, we find in Orthodoxy an appreciation of life's development as part of a natural course, an appreciation of the "stages of development" and "passages" in each person's life. But from an Orthodox perspective, attention must also be given to the process of believers' maturation in their growth toward God-likeness. The church has a definite influence on that spiritual growth and offers its own model of "mature humanity."

LIFE'S PASSAGES

The normal patterns in human life—the passage from birth through childhood, adolescence, and adulthood to aging and death—are embraced within the church's life. The Eastern Orthodox tradition has articulated its own perspective on the passages of human life, as is seen in the writings of some early church fathers.

In his commentary on the Psalms, the fourth-century church father St. Basil divides human life into three (and subsequently four) periods of seven years, which, it would appear, reflected the average life span of the people of his time. He calls these by the interesting name "weeks of years," that is, seven-year periods. If four "weeks of years" were the norm before the onset of old age, St. Basil was speaking of a life span of about

111

thirty-five years. This appears to coincide roughly with modern scholarly studies in life expectancy for the Roman Empire and Byzantium.[1] According to St. Basil, each of the stages ends with a kind of death:

> Even before the soul is divorced from the body by death, we human beings die many times. Do not think what I say is strange, but look to the truth of the thing. For each of the three weeks of years, the human being by nature is subject to changes and transformation to different ages and lives.
>
> Each week of years has its own boundary enclosing the things that are past, and manifestly providing for a transformation. The infant's age is ended with the bringing forth of permanent teeth, and is bounded by the seventh year. The child's period—appropriate for learning—has as its limit, adolescence. Until the first and twentieth year is fulfilled, when hair begins to shadow his cheeks, the age of the adolescent disappears gradually, as the young man is transformed into an adult. When therefore you see a man put away the drive for growth by age, having progressed in understanding and bearing, not a shadow of youthfulness remaining, do you not consider that all of the past has died? Again the old man, reformed in accordance to another physical shape and state of soul, is clearly different from those who went before. So it is that the life of human beings is by nature completed by means of many deaths . . . by means of the transformations of the advances in age.[2]

In another ancient work attributed to St. Basil, but not his,[3] commentary is given on the words in Genesis 1:28 understood as "increase and multiply," rather than as "be fruitful and multiply." The Septuagint word *auxanesthe* is interpreted as referring to the phased development of the human being in periods of seven years. Thus, from birth to age seven, one is an infant; from the seventh to the fourteenth year one is a child; from the fourteenth to the twenty-first one is a youth or maiden. At the twenty-first year one becomes an adult. The author opines, "thus, in the same manner we ought to advance in age [*methelikiousthe*] in every period of our lives, in accordance with each 'week of years' [*kath' ebdomadas*]." The unknown author adds, "For it says 'Increase' so that what has been created might not remain incomplete."[4]

The genuine commentary of St. Basil, using the "weeks of years" concept, focuses on the passages (the "deaths") that make each phase of life distinctive. Pseudo-Basil, using the same concept, emphasizes the fulfilling and completing character of the stages to which the passages lead. Both reflect on the process as it is experienced in the normal course of life, and both provide a traditional source of understanding for some contemporary approaches to the passages of life.

Our modern age has understood well the developmental aspects of life. Numerous disciplines have emerged to trace the development of various stages of human existence. Highly influenced by the work of psychologist Jean Piaget, researchers have formulated many different developmental theories and applied them to a wide range of human activity. For example, Lawrence Kohlberg has focused on stages of moral development,[5] and James Fowler, on stages in religious development.[6] Carol Gilligan has formulated a feminist developmental approach,[7] John Chirban has sought to integrate certain concepts in religious development with Eastern Orthodox themes,[8] and Gail Sheehy has popularized the concept of passages in general.[9]

Without doubt, these and other understandings provide valuable insights, but they are also subject to certain limitations from within the respective disciplines[10] and religious perspectives.[11] The impression given by these systems overall, despite denial by their advocates, is that the stages they describe are somehow foreordained, enclosing within them a somewhat automatic or deterministic element, even though most apologists recognize that there can be failure at any step in the process. In addition, few treatments of passages, even those that recognize religious elements, focus on the transcendent experience of passages and their liturgical embodiments in church life, together with the normative positions appropriate to each stage of life.

Given the strong liturgical tradition of Orthodox Christianity, which seeks to incorporate the whole of life into communion with God, it should not surprise us that every major passage of life is drawn into the spiritual orbit of the church by means of its worship life.

From an exclusively secular point of view, this activity of the Orthodox church may be considered a socialization process, achieved in large part by marking birth, marriage, aging, and death with ritual acts.[12] From the perspective of the church, however, there are deeper meanings for the liturgical treatment of life's passages than just the socialization process. Historically, they are intimately connected with the religious faith of Byzantium, Orthodox Christianity. These religiously inspired passage rites are illuminated by the theological presuppositions of the Orthodox faith and their embodiment in the liturgical practices of the Orthodox church, in order to sanctify life and to aid persons in community to grow into their full humanity and to achieve God-likeness. In short, the church's concern with passages is closely identified with the saving and redeeming work of Jesus Christ for all persons.

MARRIAGE AND PROCREATION

In Orthodoxy, much love is expended upon the infant, and the birth of a child is celebrated with pride and happiness. Significant rites serve to include the newborn child into the life of the Christian community: the "churching" and the baptismal service itself, and the admission of infants to the sacrament of Holy Communion. But at the head of all these is marriage and its procreative purpose.

The birth of children is seen as a blessing in the Orthodox marriage service as it is now conducted. In the Service of the Promise (formerly conducted at the time of the betrothal but now connected with the sacrament of marriage), we read: "You, O Lord, from the beginning have created male and female, and by You is a woman joined to a man for assistance and for the continuation of the human race." The text of the marriage ceremony itself is also quite specific regarding the birth of children. The initial litany invites all those present to pray "that there may be given unto them [the couple being married], soberness of life, and fruit of the womb as may be most expedient for them. . . . [13]

The main body of the service also refers to childbirth as one of the purposes of marriage. Thus the biblical command to "increase and multiply" is frequently repeated. The service even looks forward to the satisfactions the couple will experience as grandparents! "Give to them fruit of the womb, fair children, concord of soul and body. . . . Let them behold their children's children as newly planted olive trees round about their table."[14] The image of the "newly planted olive trees" must have evoked the vitality, brightness, and vigor of newly born life in familial and community environment for the unknown author of these lines.

INITIATION INTO LIFE

A series of rites and services exists to mark the beginning of the life of children born into Orthodox Christian families, though all these are not practiced extensively in the United States. They serve, even before the child has been baptized, to welcome and acknowledge the child's presence, to begin the process of integration into the faith community, and to give the child identification as an Orthodox Christian, almost as a birthright.

The traditional prebaptismal rites offered by the church for the newborn and the newborn's family consist of prayers and brief services on the first day after a woman has given birth, on the eighth day at the traditional naming of the child, and on the fortieth day at the churching of the mother and child. Formulated in the framework of village social life, these prayers are with difficulty implemented on schedule in the urban and suburban realities of America. Nevertheless, priests visit the hospitals frequently, offering the prayers for the first day of birth as soon as possible following the event. Although a few priests may also visit the home for the naming service on the eighth day or shortly thereafter, this service is probably conducted the least often.[15] The churching on the fortieth day is widespread.

Three prayers are offered at the bedside of the mother and child "On the First Day after a Woman Has Given Birth to a Child." The first is a prayer for healing and protection: "O Sovereign Master and Lord Almighty, Who heals every sickness and every weakness, do You Yourself heal this servant (Name) who this day has borne a child, and raise her up from the bed on which she lies. . . . Protect her, and this child which she has borne; shelter her under the covering of Your wings from this day to her last." The second prayer expands on the protection theme with specific reference to both bodily sickness (especially postpartum disturbances) and the spiritual ills of the new mother, as well as the health of the child. Petitions are also offered regarding the future of the child: "and of the infant which has been born of her do You account worthy to worship in the earthly temple which You have prepared for the glorification of Your Holy Name." The first expectation of the child is that it will become a member of the worshipping community of the church. The final prayer refers to the Genesis injunction to "increase and multiply" but is primarily a prayer for forgiveness of the mother, the whole household, and all those who have come in contact with her (including the midwife, the family members, and even the priest). The ascription of the dismissal prayer is to "Christ, our true God, who was born in a cave and who lay down in a stable for our salvation."[16] More will be said below about the prayers for forgiveness that are part of these rites.

The prayers for blessing of the child on the eighth day are designated by the rubrics to be offered at the "western doors" of the church building (the outside doors of the temple). The midwife, not the mother, brings the child. After blessing various parts of the child's body with the sign of the cross, the prayer of the "signing" is read. The first petition asks that the child be "signed" with the light of God's countenance in the "heart and understanding," so that the child "may flee the vanity of this wicked world and every evil device of the Enemy [the devil] and may follow your commandments, instead." The first name given to the child is the name of God: "grant, O Lord, that Your Name may remain on him (her) unrenounced, when at a fitting time he (she) shall be conjoined with Your Holy Church, and is perfected through the dread Mysteries [sacraments] of Your Christ." The vision for the life of the newborn child is not limited, however, to membership in the church on earth. The prayer asks, on the condition that God's commandments be observed and that the newborn keeps "the Seal unbroken," that the child may "attain the blessedness of Your elect in Your Kingdom." The rubrics then instruct the priest to take the child "before the gates of the temple" or before the icon of the Theotokos and to repeat a prayer to the Virgin Mother which also makes reference to Symeon, who received the Christ-child in the temple on the fortieth day (Luke 2:21–40). It is clear that this is a "next step" in the process of being brought fully into the life of the church. The child is brought to (but not into) the temple and is marked, or "signed," with the sign of the cross and with the "Name of God."

On the fortieth day after the birth of the child, custom and church rubrics call for the "churching" of the mother and the child, a tradition practiced widely in the U.S. On the fortieth day (or more likely on the Sunday following) the parents are met by the priest in the church narthex, which leads to the sanctuary proper. Standing before the open doors of the sanctuary, the priest begins by reciting several prayers that focus upon the creative work of God, offer thanksgiving for the preservation of the life of the mother, ask for forgiveness of her sins and for her physical and ritual cleansing and purification following her birth-giving. It is also asked that the mother be received back into the sacramental life of the church upon the completion of the forty days.

Prayers are also offered for the newborn child, in anticipation of the baptism: "Bless also this child which has been born of her; increase it, sanctify it, give it understanding and a prudent and virtuous mind; for You alone have brought it into being, and have shown him (her) the light which the bodily sense perceives, so that he (she) might be accounted worthy also of the ideal Light and be numbered with Your holy Flock."[17]

After several such prayers are read, the priest takes the child in his hands and enters the sanctuary. The rubrics read: "Then, taking up the child, the Priest lifts it up in the sign of the Cross before the Gates of the Temple, saying: 'The servant of God (Name) is churched, in the Name of the Father, and of the Son, and the Holy Spirit. Amen.' " This is repeated in the middle of the church and once more at the front of the sanctuary. If the child is a girl, the priest proceeds to the Royal Gates (the center doors of the icon screen that separates the sanctuary area where the laity are seated from the altar area). Standing before the open doors, the priest repeats the words of Symeon from Luke 2:29–32. If the child is a boy, the priest goes through the doors, repeats the words of Symeon, walks around the altar table, and concludes with the repetition of the words of Symeon. The priest then invites the parents forward to receive their child, now "presented" to the Lord and his church. This rite, with its clear parallels to the Presentation of Jesus in the Temple and its messianic implications, serves to initiate the child into the community, even before baptism. The difference in the ritual for boys and girls probably reflects the possibility that the boy will receive a call to the priesthood.

In any case, for all Orthodox children the churching is a preliminary step to the full theological and sacramental incorporation of the child into the body of the church through the sacraments of baptism, chrismation, and Holy Communion.

From the point of view of the health and well-being of the new mother and child, the service of the churching on the fortieth day has important significance. With this rite, the mother and the child leave the special period of life known as the *locheia* in Greek, that is, "the confinement, childbed, or lying-in" period, and now take their place in the normal course of life. The mother, in particular, in receiving this special status following birth, is also given protection. By custom, she is exempted from ordinary work; she is to rest and care for her newborn child. During the *locheia* she traditionally receives special assistance and care from her relatives, and she is not permitted to have sexual relations with her husband. She is allowed, in short, time for recuperation and the regaining of her strength. The psychological value of this period is immense, not only for herself, but also for the very important first days of nurture and care for the child. The *locheia* seeks to assure peace and a measure of solitude; it encourages a warm, caring, and intimate environment for the newborn child. Though this aspect of the tradition is in competition with the activist mores of modern society, it still serves in many ways to provide a brake on the pressures placed upon new mothers. The contemporary movement to insure maternity leaves for working mothers may well be a witness to the wisdom of this ancient church tradition.

The prayers for the forgiveness of sins related to the pregnancy or the childbirth must be carefully understood. These have to be seen in the larger context of Orthodox worship and not as a negative judgment on childbirth itself. No service of any kind in the Orthodox church omits petitions for the forgiveness of sins; thus it would be a genuine anomaly if petitions for forgiveness were absent from this service. All that is implied by these petitions is that in our fallen condition we do nothing without some measure of sinfulness, and that all the wholesome aspects of life need to be incorporated into the life of the kingdom of God. This is precisely what the churching does for the new mother and her baby.

The same needs to be understood about the passing reference to the new mother's condition of "uncleanliness." What needs to be made clear is that the "purifying" aspect of the rite refers to her bodily condition, not her ethical status. Only if one judges from a moralistic perspective not congenial to the Orthodox tradition is it possible to understand the reference as a condemnation of the birth event.

Of what, then, is the mother purified? Purification is from the biological disruption of her body as a consequence of her birth-giving. The disruption, a physiological experienced reality, cannot simply be defined out of existence. Because it is a real part of the new mother's condition, the prayers address it. The bleeding, the healing process, the readjustment of the internal organs, the beginning of lactation, and all the immense changes that take place in her body during the first month or so after birth are sufficiently completed by the fortieth day. Her body, in large measure, has returned to normal. And so it is pronounced, by her ritual return to normal social and church life. Physicians note that the uterus, for example, returns to normal functioning in about four weeks, when menstruation can begin (unless, of course, the mother is breast-feeding). Current recommendations are that sexual relations between spouses can resume about six weeks after birth. The ancient rite of churching seems to have institutionalized these medical perceptions and prescriptions.[18]

The churching service provides one more example of the way Eastern Christianity unites into a single perspective the varied dimensions of life. It is sensed as a profoundly meaningful rite that unites physical and spiritual concerns. One priest commented in writing to me: "It is wise that mother and child should be excluded from church attendance for the forty days so that they may bond. I enjoy the prayers and the presence of the mother and child in their "debut" in the life of the community. I do it with the entire congregation present on Sunday morning." Although the service is normally a private one, this priest's practice emphasizes the corporate dimension of the rite along with the spiritual and physical dimensions for an even fuller experience of wholeness.

BAPTISM, CHRISMATION, AND FIRST COMMUNION

As noted above, formal entry into the life of the church occurs at baptism. For the vast majority in the Orthodox church this is in practice a threefold liturgical rite, including the sacraments of baptism and chrismation and the first reception of Holy Communion. Whatever other theological meaning it may have, baptism here is understood as the passage *par excellence* from the "old" life of separation from God to the "new" life in the kingdom of God.

Liturgical scholar Alcibiadis C. Calivas understands baptism in a way highly reminiscent of the understanding of the "weeks of years," described above both as a sort of "death" and as a fulfillment:

> Baptism is the initial and essential mystery (i.e., sacrament) and an absolute, decisive action for the Christian. The benefits of Christ's incarnation, death and resurrection are mediated to the believer through Baptism. Baptism engraves upon and imparts to each person afresh the image of God. . . .
>
> The baptismal font becomes at once a tomb and a womb: "at the self-same moment you die and are born; the water of salvation is at once your grave and your mother" (St. Cyril of Jerusalem). The triple immersion in and emersion from the baptismal waters is laden with meaning. Baptism is both a death and a new birth. The water destroys one life and it begets another. It drowns the old man and raises up the new. The liturgical act gives expression to two realities: the death of the old man, who in solidarity with Adam, is subject to sin and death, and the birth of the new man, who in his union with Christ, is provided with new members and faculties in preparation for the time to come.

Calivas calls baptism "the beginning of a process of becoming," reflecting the theological tradition of Orthodoxy which sees growth in the image and likeness of God as a lifelong spiritual characteristic of the Christian way. Regarding "infant baptism," he notes that "such baptisms are not performed in a vacuum, but upon the explicit expression of faith by parents and sponsors, and especially the very community itself, gathered to celebrate the mystery (sacrament), each time reaffirming its faith, pledging itself to provide an environment of continued Christian witness for its members."[19] All this is made visible by the baptismal rite, which includes a ritual rejection of the devil and evil, an acceptance of Christ, and baptism by immersion in the baptismal font.

Representing the body of the faithful in a concrete and specific way at this great passage from the kingdom of the world to the kingdom of God is the sponsor, or godparent. The sponsor speaks on behalf of the child in the acceptance of Christ and receives the child physically from the font. In Orthodox canon law as well as in popular consciousness, the sponsor is thereafter considered a relative, a member of the family, and a spiritual parent to the child.

The counterpart to Western confirmation practices, chrismation, or anointing, differs from them in taking place immediately after the child is lifted up out of the baptismal font, while still in the sponsor's arms. The child is then "sealed" with the consecrated oils, with the "gift of the seal of the Holy Spirit." The anointing of chrismation "imparts to persons the energies and the gifts of the Holy Spirit."[20] It is "forward-looking," impelling the new Christian into the exercise of the faith. It should be noted that this same sacrament is used to receive converts into the Orthodox church from other Christian faiths. It serves to confirm a new beginning.

Full membership in the church is expressed through participation in the sacrament of Holy Communion. In current Orthodox practice, the child's first Holy Communion takes place at the conclusion of the baptism-chrismation (confirmation) service, from the Holy Communion reserved in a special tabernacle on the altar table. The Orthodox church holds to a practice of "closed communion," that is, only members of the Orthodox church in spiritual good standing may participate in the sacramental communion. Whatever else the sacrament of the Eucharist may mean, in the light of the present discussion, reception of the Body and Blood of Christ for the Orthodox Christian is an affirmation of his or her identity and membership in the church.[21]

Thus from the prayer on the first day of birth through a series of liturgical steps to baptism, chrismation, and first Holy Communion, the child is incorporated into the life of the Orthodox community of faith, so that the child can never remember a time in its life when it was not part of the "people of God."

· 12 ·

Passages toward Maturation

The natural course of life presents us with the concerns occupying the next phases, or "weeks of years": those of childhood and youth, the development of sexual identity and potential activity, and the choices and responsibilities of adult life. To each of these phases the Orthodox tradition contributes a distinctive perspective.

CHILDHOOD

The early introduction of children into the life of the Orthodox Christian community requires that they be nurtured and cared for if they are to realize some measure of their life potential. What are the responsibilities of parents toward their children? The primary obligation is to affirm and protect life as a gift of God.

Opposition to abortion is thus part of the early church's first teaching. One of the earliest moral instructions given to Christians, the *Letter of Barnabas* (70–100 C.E.), teaches: "Love your neighbor more than yourself. Do not kill a fetus by abortion, or commit infanticide."[1] Often in Roman society unwanted newborns were abandoned, left vulnerable to the elements or to attacks by wild animals. Some were found by unscrupulous persons who raised them to lives of prostitution or maimed them so as to use them for begging.

The church encouraged parents who could not or would not care for their children to bring them to the church so that they could be raised in orphanages.[2] These protective views still characterize the Orthodox attitude toward children. For example, the Greek Orthodox Archdiocese of North and South America proclaimed 1987 as the "Year of the Child," focusing on the abused child. The decision inspired one iconographer, George Filippakis of Woodbury, New York, to create a large icon depicting the compassionate Christ in the presence of children being abused, graphically symbolized by a crucified child.

The growing child begins to assume responsibility for him- or herself, and the canon law of the church takes up the question of an age of account-

121

ability. The minimum age for participation in holy confession or in the monastic life given in the writings of various church fathers ranges from seven to fifteen years. Thus the age of responsibility is located at the end of the first or second "week of years." This disparity is reflected in an appreciation for particular personal capacities in a canon of the Sixth Ecumenical Council, which allows that "maturity of the reasoning faculty is attained in some persons more quickly and in others more slowly. For some persons, being of an acuter and finer nature, acquire more rapidly than others the power of discerning and distinguishing what is good and what is bad."[3]

Parents have the responsibility to care for their children, and conversely children are to obey and respect their parents. The biblical injunction in Ephesians 6:1–4 still informs the general attitude of the church toward family life: "Children, obey your parents in the Lord, for this is right. 'Honor your father and mother' (this is the first commandment with a promise), 'that it may be well with you and that you may live long on the earth.' Fathers, do not provoke your children to anger, but bring them up in the discipline and instruction of the Lord." Of special interest are two patristic writings that reflect this New Testament teaching and that have had significant influence on family life in the tradition.

In one, St. John Chrysostom provides a handbook for the raising of children titled "Address on Vainglory and the Right Way for Parents to Bring Up Their Children." The handbook may be thought of as an extended commentary on the second part of the passage from Ephesians quoted above: it combines a clear sense of the direction in which the child should grow and an awareness of the child's personal dignity and developing abilities. Chrysostom displays sensitivity to the reality that either severity or laxity can provoke negative consequences for the child.[4]

St. Basil, another fourth-century church father, addressed the content of children's education more specifically. His work *Exhortation to Youths as to How They Shall Best Profit by the Writings of Pagan Authors* introduces a principle of discernment by which Christian values are used to assess secular wisdom. Its message, according to one commentator, is that "the study of the ancient writers can be valuable if a good selection is made among the works of the poets, historians and rhetoricians, and everything is excluded which could be dangerous for the souls of the students."[5] The practical effect of this approach was that mainline Orthodox Christianity encouraged an education that included the sciences and the liberal arts (although a minority—mostly monastic—always disagreed). Though Orthodox ethnic traditions vary in their emphasis on formal education, some of them place a very high value on the education of youths.[6]

A weak point in the liturgical life of the Orthodox may be the absence of a "rite of passage" for adolescents into adulthood. Because the sacrament of chrismation (confirmation) is conducted together with baptism, and Holy Communion begins at baptism in infancy, the opportunity for a conscious reaffirmation of Christian identity as a child moves into adolescence is missed. Organizations for youth and young adults in the churches and fraternal organizations in the ethnic life of Orthodox peoples seek to meet this need. In addition, some parishes in the United States are experimenting with programs and even church rites that will address this situation as younger members move toward adulthood.

SEXUAL MATURATION AS PASSAGE

Anthropologists refer to the varied observances related to arrival at physical sexual maturation, with or without the beginning of sexual activity, as "rites of passage." In most cultures sexual maturation is closely related to entry into adulthood. Whatever the specifics in any culture, the sexual maturation of boys and girls is clearly a passage from childhood to the doorstep of adulthood.

In the contemporary world, as a result of the widespread adoption of certain psychological viewpoints about human life—aided of course by the media, economic patterns, and other social forces—sex has become one of our overt central concerns and preoccupations. Other ages and times seem to have focused their public interests on political and military power, religious faith and practice, economic activity, or mere survival, but ours has somehow made sex one of its central and most public motifs. As a result, issues of sexuality demand attention in a way unfamiliar to past generations.

This has been the experience of the Orthodox church. The concern with the phenomenon of sex, biologically, socially, religiously, and ethically understood, did not escape its attention, even though it is not at the center of its worldview. The church has been aware of the potentialities for life that sexuality offers and concurrently quite sensitive to its capacity for distortion.

The wholistic perspective characteristic of the Orthodox church has been applied to human sexuality as well, and this approach has differed from that of Western Christianity in many ways. Perhaps it is most instruc-

tive to place sexuality face to face with the central concern of the church—
holiness. In that apparent confrontation, we will see in sharp outline the
distinctive Orthodox approach to sexuality.

At issue for the church is the relationship of the sexual dimensions of life
and the sanctification of life. Reconciling them has not been easy. On the
one hand, the sacrament of holy matrimony clearly shows the church's approval of marriage and marital sexual activity. But an apparently contradic-
tory message is also strongly conveyed by the powerful tradition of Eastern
Christian monasticism, with its threefold discipline of obedience, poverty,
and chastity.

Perhaps no influence on Orthodox religious life has been greater than
monasticism, the continuing reminder of the life of the kingdom of God
that ultimately transcends the institutions and concerns of "this world."
In monasticism, the ideal of chastity *means* the rejection of sexual activity. Thus, for monks, chastity is celibacy, especially when the concept
includes the whole person, body and soul, the inner and outer life. In
the Gospel of Matthew, Christ presents the ideal of celibacy to his disciples following a teaching on the permanency of the marital relationship
(Matthew 19:10–12). He offers as an alternative to marriage a willed
renunciation of all deliberate sexual activity, understood as a response to
a calling from God. God has invited some to respond to this calling as
to an offered gift. In the expectation of the imminent approach of the
kingdom, St. Paul indicated his preference that Christians remain unmarried, even as he was (1 Corinthians 7:9). He did not, however, require it of
all Christians; he commended the marriage relationship as reflecting the
relationship of Christ with the Church, one of love and deep mutuality
(Ephesians 5).

At the same time the church interpreted various biblical passages as
properly limiting sexual activity to the married life and its faithful commitment. Yet teaching about sex has not been uniform in the tradition of Eastern Orthodoxy. Positive, negative, and mixed views about sex have tended
to color the thinking, writing, and values of those speaking for the church.[7]
But it is fair to say that in Orthodoxy the views settle into two major
tendencies.

Given that much of the spiritual and theological literature of the Orthodox church was written by monastics for monastics, and given the important place of monasticism in Orthodoxy, it is not surprising that the case
for celibate Christian living is made quite strongly in the Orthodox
tradition.[8] In much of the monastic literature true holiness seems to be
connected almost exclusively with the monastic form of the Christian life,

which of course includes celibacy as a major constitutive element. Sex in marriage is more often than not perceived only as a concession to human weakness and spiritual immaturity, though notable exceptions to this view are found, as in the teachings of St. John Chrysostom.[9]

Numerous influences in our day have provoked a response to the downgrading of married life via-à-vis holiness. Certainly, a more open and wholesome view of sex in the Western world is one. Another has been the increasing understanding of the laity's role in the life of the church, and concern for their fulfillment of the Christian way of life in ordinary life. Perhaps another, in light of Orthodoxy's powerful liturgical tradition, has been the renewal of concern with personal religious experience, experience not limited to prayer but occurring in the whole range of the Christian's daily life. Eventually, these influences have led Orthodox Christians to ask also about the place of sex in their lives and to try to relate sexuality positively to the Christian life as a whole. The effort has not been exercised as a competitive deemphasis of monasticism. Rather it has been, by and large, an effort to understand the potential of marriage for the realization of "kingdom living" and to see marriage as an appropriate context for growth in sanctity and for the fulfillment of the divine image.[10]

Despite this apparent disparity, the Orthodox church's approach to sex is fundamentally in harmony with its concern for sanctity. The issue of married and unmarried clergy provides the best illustration.

The Scriptures bear evidence that some of the apostles were married men. In the early church the clergy, including bishops, were expected to be married.[11] Nevertheless, a view arose early in the history of the church that men who engaged in sexual relations with wives were somehow not worthy to approach the holy altar. At a council held around the year 345 in Gangra in Paphlagonia, a Black Sea province in Asia Minor, these views were strongly opposed. Canon 4 says, "If anyone discriminates against a married Presbyter [priest], on the ground that he ought not to partake of the offering when that Presbyter is conducting the Liturgy, let him be anathema," that is, let him be expelled from the church.[12]

The tendency to regard marriage and priesthood as incongruent, however, remained alive, especially in the Western regions of the church under Rome. There, the idea of the priesthood's special sanctity gained favor, and marital sexual activity by priests came to be thought of as inappropriate. Clerical celibacy was slowly introduced in the West.[13]

This was not the case in the East. The status of the married priest, including his sexual activity, was defended in conscious contrast to the Western practice in the thirteenth canon of the Sixth Ecumenical Council, held in Constantinople in 691. The canon is quite instructive because it also sheds light on limitations to sexual activity as well:

> We have learned that in the church of the Romans it is regarded as tantamount to a canon that ordinands to the deaconry or presbytery must solemnly promise to have no further intercourse with their wives. Continuing, however, in conformity with the ancient canon of apostolic rigorism and orderliness, we desire that henceforward the lawful marriage ties of sacred men become stronger, and we are nowise dissolving their intercourse with their wives, nor depriving them of their mutual relationship and companionship when properly maintained in due season, so that if anyone is found to be worthy to be ordained a Subdeacon, or a Deacon, or a Presbyter, let him nowise be prevented from being elevated to such a rank while cohabitating with a lawful wife. Nor must he be required at the time of ordination to refrain from lawful intercourse with his own wife, lest we be forced to be downright scornful of marriage, which was instituted by God and blessed by his presence.[14]

Thus Eastern Christianity rejects the view that there is a fundamental incongruity between the married state and the condition of priestly service. Lawful sexual activity and the Christian life are not incompatible.

Nevertheless, the canon reflects some measure of the contradiction between the passions of sexual activity—even when legitimate—and the striving after holiness. Canon 13 continues:

> We are cognizant, though, that those who met in Carthage and made provision of decency in the life of clergy declared that Subdeacons and Deacons and Presbyters, busying themselves as they do with the sacred mysteries, according to their rules, are obliged to practice temperance in connection with their helpmates, in order that we may likewise keep the injunction handed down by the Apostles, and continued from ancient times in force, well knowing that there is a proper season for everything, and especially for fasting and praying. For those who assist in the ceremonies at the sacrificial altar have to be temperate in all things at the time when they are handling holy things, so that they may be able to gain whatever they ask for.[15]

In practice, this means that Orthodox priests are to avoid sexual contact with their wives on the night before they conduct the Divine Liturgy and on the day following it, and during fast periods. Among laypeople, it is expected that sexual activity be avoided in particular during the preparation period before receiving Holy Communion. The message is that sex is subservient to sanctity. Yet sex may be a vehicle for holy purposes as well, expressing within the context of marriage a vision of the kingdom and the bond of unity, the trinitarian reality of love.

The absolute rejection of sexual activity by monastics and the acceptance of married sexual activity at appropriate times by deacons and priests point to an aspect of Eastern Orthodoxy's approach to the question of sex and sanctity summarized in 1 Corinthians 7:7. St. Paul says, "I wish that all were as I myself am [celibate]. But each has his own special gift from God, one of one kind and one of another." Some "have a gift from God," a calling to a life that renounces sexual activity; more have a gift from God lawfully and legitimately to express their sexual reality in marriage. Each may use the sexual dimension of what he or she is by placing it in the service of God. This very approach, by placing sexuality within the life of the kingdom, calls for its transformation.

The celibate road is not so much a denial of sexuality as its transfiguration and a consecration. Since in the eschatological eternal kingdom there is no "marrying or giving in marriage" but life is like that of "angels in heaven" (Matthew 22:30), the monastic life (together with the life of total obedience and poverty) is a fuller earthly manifestation of heavenly life. Consequently, it is honored more than the married life in Orthodoxy. Nevertheless, the married life is, as we have seen, not condemned nor considered unholy but is highly honored.

In any case, both the monastic and the marital ways are "gifts" and "callings" within the new life. Both in their own way may point to the life of the kingdom. Both are to be transfigured in the light of Christ. Otherwise both are worldly conditions. Purity ought to characterize them both. Both, imbued by the Spirit of God, are expressions of God-likeness in service and in love.

Visibly, the account of the Transfiguration of Christ and the icon presented to the faithful illustrate this truth dramatically. The transfigured Christ is seen with two Old Testament personages, Moses and Elijah (Elias). Moses was married; Elias was celibate. Both share in the illumination revealing the light and brilliance of the divine. Each, with his own gift and calling, responds in worship and adoration in communion with the transfiguring light of God. Sexuality comes into its own, as is the case with every aspect of life, when brought into communion with God.[16]

MARRIAGE

Although the Orthodox church understands marriage as a sacrament, church teaching also recognizes marriage as a universal human institution. The Genesis accounts emphasize both the procreative purpose and the unitive, companionate, supportive qualities of marriage.[17] Some interpretations of the sacramental character of marriage emphasize its bestowal of blessings upon the couple.[18] Unquestionably, some of the prayers in the contemporary marriage service support the view that the sacrament of marriage intends to convey the presence of the Holy Spirit to the shared life of the couple.

But contemporary Orthodox theologians of marriage tend to understand the sacrament as primarily introducing the natural (yet fallen) relationship of marriage into the fulfilled realm of the kingdom of God. The sacrament provides a vision of a full and complete marital relationship precisely because it is related to God and his kingdom. A modern Greek writer puts it this way:

> Marriage is a way of life, a dynamic expression of freely given love, a call of a specific human being, of the man or the woman, to travel the way of perfection or theosis. It is a way by which a person makes real his grace-filled and prophetic this-worldly presence and responsibility. *Thus marriage is not a closed or individualistic mode of life, but rather, it is a potential for us to realize in substance and practice that which we ought to become, being fully enflamed by love.*[19]

Thus the meaning of marriage as a sacrament transcends any of its given purposes. It is in marriage that the vast majority of believers will seek to manifest their own humanity as persons growing in the image and likeness of God, or as the Orthodox say, "toward theosis." There individualism and self-centeredness may be overcome in the intimate community of two persons, reflecting the life of the persons of the Holy Trinity—one in essence yet a plurality of persons in communion. Marriage as a sacrament relates the human and the divine.

Over the centuries a separate and impressive rite emerged.[20] It consists of two parts: the Service of the Promise, involving the blessing of the couple and the exchange of rings, and the Service of the Crowning, in which the crowning of the couple is a sign of their new responsibility, dignity, and place in society as the heads of a new household.[21] The rings represent the couple's promises to take each other as spouse and to remain faithful and true. They are exchanged three times to emphasize the mutuality of the commitment. The crowns likewise are exchanged three times, with the groom's crown touching the bride's head and the bride's crown touching the head of the groom, again emphasizing the mutuality of the relationship. In its litanies, prayers, and liturgy the service presents a complex of expectations and purposes for marriage in the church: mutual commitment to the life of salvation; the procreation of children; a unity of understanding, decision making, and life-purposes based on a common religious faith and experience; a deeply realized personal communion and shared trust; absolute faithfulness to each other and to their marriage; the assumption of the couple's place within the social fabric; a sexual life free of sin and reflective of their unity as spouses.

The wholeness of these goals is perceived as being realized in the vision of the kingdom of God and as a result of the blessing of God. It is neither the couple who brings the marriage about nor the officiating priest. Rather, as the most ancient of the prayers indicates, it is God: "do You Yourself, O Sovereign Lord, stretch forth Your hand from Your holy dwelling place, and join together this Your servant (name) and Your servant (name), for by You is a wife joined to her husband."[22]

In marriage and family life, just as in all aspects of the practical life of the church, the kingdom vision provides a standard toward which Christians are called to grow. Yet the very character of this approach implies that marriages and families do not reach the ideal instantaneously. To grow toward these goals requires much effort and much divine grace, and no marriage achieves them fully. In what might justifiably be called "successful marriages" the process is fulfilled slowly, with much attention to relationships and with the sharing of both joys and happinesses as well as sorrows, difficulties, and failures.

But the Orthodox church does not ignore the breakup and dissolution of marriages. It is true that the first marriage remains the ideal one; no second marriage, whatever its cause, is honored as much as the first, which is placed in an eternal framework. The church nevertheless blesses second and third marriages of widowed persons and also allows some persons civilly divorced to be remarried in the church a second or third time.[23] Remarriages are conducted as an expression of compassion and merciful pastoral concern for the spiritual well-being of the believer. An essential part of the ecclesiastical divorce proceedings is the church's concerted effort to effect a reconciliation; only certain conditions are admitted as justifying the granting of an ecclesiastical divorce.[24]

FAMILY LIFE AND SINGLE ADULTHOOD

The year 1987 was proclaimed the "Year of the Family" in the Greek Orthodox Archdiocese of North and South America. The decision to do so was provoked by concern for the breakdown of family life in the nation and in the church, as indicated by increasing divorce rates, the radical increase in the number of "mixed marriages" over the past two decades, and the rapid dissolution of the extended ethnic family structure.

As of this writing, in some Orthodox church jurisdictions in the United States 60–70 percent of the marriages are between Orthodox Christians and non-Orthodox Christians. According to Orthodox practice, such marriages must take place in the Orthodox church in order to assure sacramental communion to the Orthodox member. When it does not, the Orthodox member is no longer "in good order." He or she may not receive Holy Communion, may not be a sponsor in a baptism or wedding, and may not hold office in the parish council. Membership in the church, consequently, though not abolished, is curtailed. Marriages are not performed in the Orthodox church between members and non-Christians.[25]

When children are born, the sacrament of baptism is the means not only to incorporate them into the life of the church as individuals but also to admit them into the life of the community and the extended family as well. Where families observe such traditions as setting up an icon shrine, fasting, celebrating church feasts, receiving Holy Communion as a family, attending church regularly, and participating in the life of the local parish, a wholesome integration of the family into the life of the church takes place. Religious education and activities for youth seek to retain loyalty and commitment to church values in young people. Typical is the Young Adult League of the Greek Orthodox Archdiocese, which focuses on a fourfold vision: *leitourgia* (worship), *martyria* (witness), *diakonia* (service), and *koinonia* (community).

How do single adults fit into Orthodox church life? This becomes more of an issue as marriages in our society take place later and later in life. Contemporary society proclaims in a thousand ways that sexual expression is an absolute necessity for all persons, whether married or unmarried. Facing this is the biblically rooted teaching of sexual purity before marriage and the traditional understanding of sexual relations before marriage as sinful. For those who understand what they have done as sin, there is repentance and forgiveness in the sacrament of holy confession. But for many Christians who seek to live the Christian life, a dilemma remains.

Historically, the church has responded by pointing to an ideal of consecrated singleness. The Scriptures and the early church recognized a class of persons who were neither clergy nor monks yet who lived lives of consecration "in the world." They were the widows, who though previously married now devoted their lives to the church and its work, and the virgins, who lived lives of sexual purity. As improbable as it may seem to many in this era, there are still among the Orthodox what may be called "committed singles" who live their lives in the world, but without any overt genital sexual expression. They live in service to others (usually relatives), to society, and to the church. Within this class, the Orthodox community recognizes the special sanctity of the *kosmokalogeros*, the "monastic living in the world." Through their particular pattern of living they also point to the life of the kingdom of God, affirming that sexuality is to be perceived as within the context of kingdom living and not the other way around.[26]

This chapter illustrates the Orthodox church's concern for the health and well-being of human beings created for God-likeness. The tradition encompasses the life of the believer at every stage, seeking to establish communion with the saving and sanctifying life of the kingdom of God. Movement through each of the "weeks of years" from birth to childhood to adulthood—especially as it is influenced by sexual maturation, gender, and the varied choices that adulthood presents—is clearly a process shared by the whole of humanity. The difference for the church is that each of these passages is perceived not only in itself but in the light of the Christian worldview.

Concern with life transitions serves to illustrate the main theme of this book: that the Eastern Orthodox tradition places not only health and medicine but all aspects of life in a spiritual context. That very concern, however, provokes other questions. Toward what goal should this growth move? This question provokes at last a vision of the realization of full humanity in each person, the topic of the next chapter. Because the answer is of necessity cast ultimately in terms of what human beings "ought to be," that is, in an ethical mode, we will be looking at a vision that is still forming Orthodox consciousness.

· 13 ·

Maturity and Development

The Orthodox vision for human life, unlike the secular "human potential" movements so popular today, is not focused exclusively on our individual abilities, nor does it rest on a static understanding of human nature. Rather, it is based on the two poles of God and the truth that all human beings have been created in the image of God and are called to realize the likeness of God in their lives. The first section of this chapter, then, deals with the meaning of spiritual and theological maturity.

Paradoxically, however, this perspective also allows for a development of understanding of the very nature of that humanity; it may challenge older understandings and allow for creative responses to new situations. An example of a deepening understanding of old perspectives is the developing teachings regarding women in the Orthodox church, the subject of the second section of this chapter. Finally, the application of the vision of human life as God-likeness to new situations will be illustrated by a sketch of emerging Eastern Orthodox views on bioethical issues.

MATURE ADULTHOOD

The doctrine of divinization, or theosis, is at the heart of the Orthodox religious life, its liturgical practices, its spirituality, and its ethic.[1] A major aspect of this doctrine is growth in the divine image. Without question, that growth occurs primarily in the spiritual and ethical dimension of the Christian life, and in some sense it is not rigidly tied to the normal developmental patterns of all human existence. Nevertheless, each stage of life has its appropriate and fitting moral obligations and spirituality.

The biblical passage that best summarizes this view is found in the letter to the Ephesians; there St. Paul talks about the church and its work, which exists "for the equipment of the saints, for the work of ministry, for the building up of the body of Christ, until we all attain to the unity of the faith and of the knowledge of the Son of God, to mature manhood, to the measure of the fullness of Christ; so that we may no longer be children" (Ephesians 4:12–14). These attainments may well have little to do with chronological age, as the lives of numerous youthful saints attest. An example is the brilliant, intelligent, virtuous, and spiritually well-rounded St. Katherine of Alexandria, who is presented in the tradition as more than a match for the intelligentsia of fourth-century Alexandria.[2]

But education and sophistication are not essential to developing the God-like life, as shown by the class of saints known as the neomartyrs. During the four hundred years of Ottoman lordship over the Orthodox peoples of Southern Europe, Palestine, and Egypt, ordinary folk were frequently challenged either to deny Christ and accept Islam or to suffer horrendous tortures and death. An example is the story of a cook, Ephrosynos, whose otherwise common life was challenged by a demand that he apostasize from the faith. His refusal cost him his life.[3]

It is not desirable to sketch a rigid "ideal type" of Christian; we need look only at the model of Christ himself and the saints. The chief means for realizing a "mature humanity" in God-likeness is participation in the life of the church. A summary statement comes from a contemporary effort to explicate the biblical injunction (2 Peter 1:4) that human beings are to become partakers of divine nature:

> The road toward Theosis, our union with God, can be formulated in the following short statement: divine grace and human freedom; theory and action; enthusiastic zeal and deliberate decision; abandonment of the "world" (meaning "sin") and return to God; good works as a means toward Theosis; a warm heart and vigilant eye. We *are* able to walk that road. We will be accompanied and strengthened by divine grace. The Holy Mysteries (sacraments) are what transmit this grace of the All-Holy Spirit. His sanctifying and deifying energy is actualized in the holy services of the Church, especially in holy Baptism, Repentance and the Divine Eucharist. It is fulfilled and completed with prayer and love.[4]

In Orthodoxy "God-likeness" has been frequently summarized in the terms *freedom* and *love*. For the Orthodox tradition, freedom (*eleutheria*) is not understood as "doing anything one pleases." Rather it means coming to a state in which one lives without disharmony or conflict with his or her divine-like nature. Such coincidence exists between the subjective self-understanding and the image and likeness of God in the person that choices, actions, and words simply flow uninhibitedly in an ever-increasing manifestation of God-like life. That this manifestation is not self-centered and confined to individual life is seen in the tradition's focus on *agape* love. The model for love is the life of the Holy Trinity. The three persons of the Holy Trinity exist in loving, interpenetrating, and mutually fulfilling love. The doctrine of the Trinity declares that one cannot be a person without loving and that a person cannot be God-like without loving. For the Orthodox, this is the description of full and "God-like" humanity.[5] Freedom and love, then, combine in a movement toward the fulfillment of the divinely given potential in every human being. As we seek to make God-likeness a reality in the specific situations of our lives, we are continually called to "self-determination" (in Greek, not *eleutheria* but *autexousion*). In the self-determining process toward God-likeness, it is understood that the choices made bear fruit only in conjunction with the guiding, strengthening, enlightening, and empowering presence and energies of God, that is, divine grace. The Orthodox call this *synergy*—the cooperation of human efforts with the leading presence of God in their lives.

James W. Fowler, an expert in the field of faith development, takes note of this Orthodox approach to the process of spiritual maturation in his book *Becoming Adult, Becoming Christian:*

> The Christian approach to the transformation from self-groundedness to vocational existence involves, then, the affirmation of *both* development and conversion. The spiritual traditions of the Eastern Orthodox branch [*sic*] of the Christian community have a special way of describing the process of ongoing conversion by which God rectifies and realigns human development. They speak of the gracious gift of divine "synergy" working with and bringing to wholeness and completion our potentials and their development. Synergy means cauterization and healing of our tendencies to self-groundedness. Synergy means the mingling of divine love with our capacities to love, guiding them and grounding them in the grace of God. Synergy means the release of a quality of creativity and energy that manifests our likeness to the restored image of God in us. Synergy means human beings fully alive and using the gift of our strengths and virtues in the service of the realization of the commonwealth of love. . . . [I]n our present situation of confusion and ferment regarding images of human wholeness and completion, we are in *critical* need of a theory of transformation and development that takes account of the power and availability to us of the synergy of God's grace.[6]

With the exception of some implications of the final sentence of this paragraph, the perspective presented is fully in harmony with the Orthodox approach to human maturation.[7]

This exposition, however, harbors a danger: it tends to focus the mind exclusively on the individual. There is a vast difference between modern individualism and the Orthodox approach. Love is one of the major elements of God-likeness precisely because God is a trinity of persons perpetually related to one another in love. Yet God is not content to remain closed within his own, albeit trinitarian, nature. A fundamental characteristic of God is to reach out from his own nature through his divine energies, to create, to sustain what he has created, to redeem it, save it, and ultimately to include it in his kingdom.

This model of involvement with the world points to what might be called the corporate, even organic relationship of the mature personality with others. This can be readily illustrated by a few comments on Romans 12, in which St. Paul deals with the corporate character of the Christian life: "I bid every one among you not to think of himself more highly than he ought to think, but to think with sober judgment, each according to the measure of faith which God has assigned him." Although much of modern life in a Western, technologically oriented society focuses on individual rights and maintains as a supreme value the appeal to justice, St. Paul's vision regards other values as having greater significance. Certainly Eastern Orthodoxy does not ignore the individual person, nor human rights, nor issues of justice. But these values do not dominate its understanding of human maturity.

St. Paul teaches that each person has gifts—in different measure and in different kind—that are needed by others. Thus the text continues: "For as in one body we have many members, and all the members do not have the same function, so we, though many, are one body in Christ, and individually members one of another" (verses 4–5). This is neither a theological nicety nor a doctrinal abstraction. It is at the core of adult and mature personhood in the Orthodox perspective. Maturity realizes itself in communion with God ("the measure of faith") and in the mutuality of the body of Christ. It focuses on what we *give*, rather than on what we get, in the image and likeness of our gracious God. Paul continues, "Having gifts that differ according to the grace given to us, let us use them. . . . " Verses 6–8 enumerate these gifts—prophecy, service, teaching, exhortation, contributions, helpfulness, and mercy—all of which are clearly directed not to self but to others.

There follows one of many lists of virtues in the Pauline writings that give a vignette of Christian character and mature adulthood. Included are love, fighting against evil, mutual support and respect, enthusiasm, living as God's servant, joyousness, patient bearing of difficulties, praying persistently, being both philanthropic and hospitable. In relation to those who persecute, the mature bless and do not speak evil of them. They are sensitive to others, rejoicing with the happy and empathetically relating to those who seek to "overcome evil with good" (Romans 12:9–21).

Such a description of Christian maturity contrasts strikingly with the individualism of our day and with our decidedly legal focus on rights and justice. Although working for rights and justice (especially for oppressed others, but also for one's self in specific situations) is sometimes the most mature course, this passage clearly indicates that the thrust of human maturity is in mutual service, in using one's gifts in a gracious way for others and graciously accepting the gifts of others in one's own life.

Given perspectives that focus on corporateness and mutuality, we might expect that the Orthodox norms for human beings growing toward "Godlikeness" would be in some ways "out of step" with contemporary standards. Nevertheless, the very understanding of human maturity is subject to expansion and development in Orthodox Christianity. A case in point is the development of Orthodox views regarding women: in this area historical conditioning has inhibited the full flowering of foundational Orthodox teaching regarding mature human living.

DEVELOPING TEACHINGS ABOUT WOMEN

In some ways the church's proclamation of its beliefs, when articulated as theological principle, can be seen as an unchanging given. But the practical implementation of the faith teachings may vary from generation to generation depending on the current context.[8] A case in point is the place of women in the church and the assessment of the status of women in general. Much of the patristic writing on women is colored by the monastic commitment to celibacy and a consequent, though not necessary, negative relationship of monks toward women. This is a function of the attitude of many of the church fathers toward the human condition and gender differences in particular. On the theological level, an equality between men and women is acknowledged. But negative attitudes also abound in regard to women. Often this seems a kind of psychological "transference" or "projection" of personal struggles onto women in general. This is especially seen in the literature of the church that expresses the problems and interests of its monastic community.

By being selective in choosing patristic passages, one could illustrate a view that women are "inferior," "the cause of human sin," "weak," "unintelligent," and so on. Conversely, one could also "prove" the "superiority," "goodness," and "excellence" of women from the patristic writings. The juxtaposition of Eve and Mary often becomes the occasion for such assessments of women in the tradition. Serious errors in assessing the tradition can be made by ignoring the rhetorical character of much of this writing and by treating it selectively in a polemical fashion.[9] A more general appreciation of Christian relationships between the church fathers and pious and devoted Christian women provides material for a more wholesome and less strident assessment of the situation.

In the twentieth century the climate of feminism is not absent from the Orthodox church, but for the reasons given above it is for the most part more muted than in other churches. This is also true in reference to the question of ordaining women. The Orthodox church is officially opposed to the idea of ordaining women to the priesthood. Many, however, believe that the ancient tradition of having deaconesses needs to be revived. The liturgical function of deaconesses is debated today, but all agree that the institution of deaconesses primarily served important pastoral needs in the life of the early church. Orthodox theologian Kyriaki FitzGerald has recently made a strong case for reintroducing the order of deaconesses.[10] Resistance comes from several quarters, not least from what might be called an antifemale bias in some traditions of Orthodox monasticism. In addition, the cultural tradition of the Roman *pater familias* has continued in ethnic and cultural practice to the present day.

Nevertheless, other forces present in the tradition make resistance to a larger place for women in the church increasingly inappropriate. The Gospels present Jesus as possessing an essential respect for the dignity and humanity of women. We find no evidence of antifeminine prejudices in his words or deeds. The early church saw the saving work of Jesus Christ as equally applicable to both men and women. For St. Paul the baptismal experience fundamentally unites all people in Christ: "For as many of you as were baptized into Christ have put on Christ. There is neither slave nor free, there is neither male nor female: for you are all one in Christ Jesus" (Galatians 3:27–28). The point is not that slaves cease to be slaves and that masters cease to be masters, or that the gender of baptized Christians is ignored or disappears, but rather that as Christians stand before God, their salvation in Christ and common humanity forms a new basis for their relationship with others. Cast in the spirit of mutuality dominant in the Eastern Christian understanding of human maturity, the relationships of men and women are not seen normatively as competing or antagonistic. Christians serve with the gifts given by God to each, and each serves in his or her own way. Nevertheless, they share in a common, redeemed humanity, each with a potential for full God-likeness. Consequently, dominance, subjugation, power, and exploitation ought not characterize relationships between men and women.

Clement of Alexandria, writing at the end of the second century, demolished the idea of the double standard of morality for Christians in his book *The Instructor:* "The virtue of men and women is the same," he wrote.[11] St. Gregory of Nazianzus wrote that his mother assumed a leadership role in her household, influencing her husband:

> she who was given by God to my father became not only, as is less wonderful, his assistant, but even his leader, drawing him on by her influence in deed and word to the highest excellence. . . . She is a woman who while others have been honored and extolled for natural and artificial beauty, has acknowledged but one kind of beauty, that of the soul, and the preservation, or the restoration as far as possible, of the Divine image.[12]

It is possible to trace in civil law, moral teaching, practical tradition, and custom the unfolding implications of this revolutionary Christian affirmation of men's and women's essential humanity before God. Where previously men looked upon women first as sexual objects of an inferior order, to be used for male gratification and as "machines" for the production of legitimate offspring, now women are to be seen by them as persons who stand with equal human dignity before God, because of their creation in the image and likeness of God and in the light of the saving work of Christ. It has taken a long time for this inherent equal human dignity to become accepted and embodied consciously in our ways of living in the Orthodox church. The Orthodox are still far from fully realizing its potential.[13] Yet what it means essentially, especially from a male perspective, is that every woman with whom one comes in contact is first and above all a human being, a person in her own right, entitled to dignity, respect, honor, and equal treatment as a person created, redeemed, and sanctified by God.[14]

Recent examples of development in the Orthodox church in the United States are the essentially unchallenged acceptance of women for study in the major Orthodox theological schools (which were previously exclusively male student bodies), the ready acceptance of women as members of parish councils, and their election to offices. Unresolved issues remain, of course. But more and more the essential emphasis on the mutual dignity of men and women is being recognized in Orthodox practice.

DEVELOPING POSITIONS IN ORTHODOX BIOETHICS

The rapid and revolutionary biomedical advances of our day demand new thinking about human decision making, values, and potentials. Almost daily new ethical problems are being created, and we have no ready solutions. For the Orthodox, with their reliance on the biblical and patristic tradition, this new reality requires a mode of decision making not frequently met in the past.

It means drawing creatively on the tradition of faith. It requires a sense of the spirit and ethos of the deposit of faith, rather than a mind-set that recognizes only repetition. A searching from within for values and parallels between old and new situations is necessary. All decision making in Orthodoxy is rooted in the tradition of faith—that is, its doctrine, ethical teaching, liturgical life, and its canon law, as embodied in the church's history—and aspects of that tradition can be drawn upon in many combinations for the purpose of bioethical decision making. The process itself is a creative act, full of hazards, and there is no guarantee that anyone assuming the task will do so properly or adequately. That is why the ethicist seeking to articulate an Orthodox Christian framework for bioethics should be prepared to have his or her conclusions challenged and corrected by the same "mind of the church" that is the source for the ethical work being done. As with every aspect of the life of the Orthodox church, decision making must be understood as an ecclesial process.

The field of bioethics is still quite young, and there is no pan-Orthodox official position on many of its topics.[15] Still, it is possible, I believe, to describe several positions that will reflect general Orthodox Christian attitudes toward bioethical questions. These positions are based, of course, on the whole of the Orthodox Christian tradition. In addition, many bioethical questions—those regarding biological life, its propagation and preservation—must be considered from the perspective of Orthodoxy's established ethical tradition regarding sexuality. Two examples are conception control and sterilization. A description of the thought processes related to these two issues shows how the interplay of traditional values can change a previously accepted position.

As we saw in Chapter 12, the Orthodox church understands human sexuality as properly fulfilled only within the context of marriage. Sexual union (and the procreation of children) is only one of the purposes of marriage, along with mutual commitment and love, mutual support, and growth in harmony and unity. All these purposes are understood sacramentally; they are embraced within the life of faith. Sexual relations between spouses, therefore, are in principle good: as the marriage service puts it, "the bed is undefiled," since Christ "by His presence in Cana of Galilee declared marriage to be honorable. . . ."[16] Certainly such meaning cannot be attributed to casual sexual behaviors that are not equally open to all the other purposes of marriage. The church must therefore also deal with the issues of *sexual sin*.

The whole range of behaviors that constitute the so-called sexual revolution in the twentieth century is perceived by the church as a perversion of how things ought to be. Any believer's violation of this approach to the Christian life-style is seen by the church as sinful, a distortion of sexual relations appropriately expressed in Christian life. Those who have even the slightest connection with the church know its teaching and its expectations. Given the nonlegalistic approach of Eastern Orthodoxy to sin (perceived less as a violation of rules than as a breaking of the appropriate relationship between ourselves and God), guilt is not at the center of the response to these and other sins. Rather, the sense of disappointment, even shame, predominates, for sin is more a failure, a disappointment, even an insult to God, distorting and violating the fitting relation between a Christian and his or her Lord.[17]

In the mind of the church, neither fornication, nor "living together," nor adulterous relations, nor masturbation, nor homosexual unions, nor pornography, nor the pansexualism of contemporary society can fulfill the genuine purpose of sex within the larger context of human life, whose goal is to reflect kingdom life in the here and now. At the heart of this ethical stance is recognition that the family is an essential moral, spiritual, and social foundation of human life and that it must be preserved and strengthened.[18] The church knows that many fall into sexual sins, and it calls for repentance and renewal of life for those who commit them. It does this through the sacrament of holy confession. Those disengaged from the life of prayer, worship, and conscious Christian living may not heed the call to repentance. Those who seek to live a life in harmony with their potential for God-likeness struggle in their daily life to avoid sin. When they sin, they seek out forgiveness and renewal. This, then, is the framework for considering the bioethical issues involved in propagating and preserving life.

The tradition's clear early teaching against abortion (witnessed in church documents of the second and third centuries and its canon law to the present day) should not be confused with the conception control issue.[19] The issue of the *prevention of conception* through so-called birth-control practices is dealt with in the patristic tradition, but on several different levels. As a result, contemporary Orthodox Christianity contains varied views on the subject.[20] When the issue was first debated in the first half of the twentieth century, the general approach was to draw on Western

Christian views, both Roman Catholic and Protestant; these tended to be negative in their evaluation of the morality of contraception.[21]

However, as Orthodox writers sought to draw on the theological perspectives of the church regarding sex and marriage, especially with the increased recognition of the interpersonal values of human life implied in the doctrine of growth in the image and likeness of the trinitarian God, a more flexible view came into prominence. This view holds that since one of the purposes of marriage is the procreation of children, no couple should enter into marriage without being open, in general, to having a family. To exclude the possibility of eventually having children is seen as a violation of their calling to live their Christian lives as married persons. Nevertheless, this newer position does not focus upon every sexual act but on the total marital relationship. Just as the petition in the marriage ceremony asks that the couple be granted children "as is expedient," so it is held that a careful use of conception control methods for the spacing of children and for the enhancement of the loving unity of the couple does not violate the purposes of marriage and may positively help in their fulfillment.[22]

Those who disagree point to patristic passages which from the contemporary vantage point seem to speak against birth-control measures but which in fact reflect mistaken views in Greek and Byzantine medicine about the process of conception. This confusion caused arguments against abortion to be understood as arguments against contraception.[23] All Orthodox theologians and moral teachers are agreed on the moral error of abortion. If birth control methods are, in fact, forms of abortion, they are to be rejected. But most are not; they, in fact, prevent conception. By careful discernment of how the tradition used certain concepts, creative new understandings have come into being in the Orthodox church.

The church's position on sterilization presents another example of that process. Those who seek sterilization usually have had children and make the decision not to have more, even though they plan to continue sexual marital relations. Their motive may be to protect the health of the mother or simply to eliminate an inhibiting factor from the unifying function of their sexual relations. A case can be made for either argument.

Nevertheless, the sense that this is a "mutilating" akin to the creation of ancient eunuchs through castration dominates normative Orthodox ethical reflection on this issue. It is interesting that one of the ancient canons prohibiting castration judges it the moral equivalent of murder, in that the potentiality for further life transmission is ended. Interestingly, the canon specifically excludes from such condemnation a castration that takes place for medical reasons.[24] It would appear that sterilization is opposed in the church because it reduces the fullness of the psychosomatic wholeness of persons, deliberately "killing" the generative dimension of human existence. It is interesting, further, to note that monks are also condemned if they castrate themselves so as not to be bothered by sexual desire. The church wants them to overcome their passionate desires through spiritual discipline as an aspect of growth in communion with God. The wholeness of our physical existence is God-given and—except for the case of life-threatening illness—ought to be preserved.

By extension, the Orthodox church tends to disapprove procedures that break up the psychosomatic wholeness of all aspects of procreation. Here Orthodox thinking is not unanimous or, for that matter, fully formed on specific issues. In the United States, however, not much concrete opposition has appeared in the Orthodox community regarding the positions that follow. Artificial insemination by donor (A.I.D.) is generally considered to be an intrusion into the spiritual and bodily unity of a married couple, a moral equivalent to adultery which is inappropriate to the wholistic vision of the marital relationship. In contrast, artificial insemination by husband (A.I.H.) tends to be perceived as a therapeutic procedure that helps a marriage achieve one of its goals.[25] For similar reasons artificial insemination of single women would not be harmonious with the wholistic vision of life in the Orthodox church.[26] Clearly the governing value is not merely what is physically "natural"; there is no sense that the use of medical technology is in itself an unwarranted intervention. Rather, it is the full unity of soul and body of the married couple that governs the Orthodox mind-set on these matters.

One would find among most Orthodox believers an almost instinctual abhorrence for practices like surrogate parenting, which is seen to destroy the wholeness of child-bearing—pairing, loving, conceiving, nurturing, birthing. For the same reason, artificial wombs and other technological wonders that foster the view of baby-making as a medicotechnical process, rather than as an expression of the shared love of a husband and wife with its spiritual, moral, psychological, and physical integrity, find no resonance in the Orthodox mind-set and ethos. For the Orthodox, parenthood, and particularly motherhood, is a high calling; it is seen as cooperation with God in the "making" of a fully developed, mature human being.

Genetic counseling and screening could in principle be supported by the Orthodox church, since "what is more or less crudely effected through the Church's rules regarding prohibited marriages because of consanguinity would be accomplished more accurately through scientific genetic screening."[27] What would not be acceptable is recourse to abortion, should it be determined by amniocentesis that a fetus was the carrier of a genetic disease.[28]

Orthodox writers have in the past frequently regarded *venereal diseases* as the unfortunate consequence of life-styles perceived to be in themselves immoral and incompatible with the Christian way of life. Though some church representatives have assumed a prophetic stance of "righteous condemnation" toward such illnesses, the emerging pattern of response is to note the association of such diseases with immoral behavior, while maintaining a compassionate approach to suffering fellow human beings. A similar approach has characterized Orthodox approaches to the phenomenon of AIDS (acquired immunodeficiency syndrome). Orthodox who have dealt with the AIDS question have sought to understand the illness but also to see its connection with life-styles that the church has always regarded as sinful (heterosexual promiscuity, homosexual practice, the use of intravenous drugs, and a hedonistic worldview). They are not impressed with the success-potential of current propaganda concerning condom use as an AIDS preventative and would prefer to work toward "risk elimination" than "risk reduction," by the restoring of proper moral standards to our society.

In July 1988 the Greek Orthodox Archdiocese of North and South America held its twenty-ninth Biennial Clergy-Laity Congress in Boston. One of the highlights of the congress was a seminar on AIDS which attracted over a thousand attendees and visitors. The session lasted for three hours, twice as long as scheduled, with much active participation by those present. The panelists included a professor of medicine, a pastoral counselor, the chair of the Orthodox Christian Association of Medicine, Psychology and Religion, a professor of Orthodox Christian ethics, and a government official from the Department of Health and Human Services, with the director of the Department of Church and Society of the archdiocese serving as moderator.[29] Nearly all the participants spoke of what might be called the "sin connection" responsible in large part for the spread of the disease. This perspective did not, however, deflect the strong philanthropic currents. Compassion for those who suffer from AIDS was an integral part of the ethos of this seminar, and support for continued research to find the means to limit the impact of the illness or to cure it was repeatedly voiced. Many of those attending agreed that such a session at a Clergy-Laity Congress a few years earlier would have been inconceivable because it would have been "too controversial" and perhaps embarrassing. In 1988, this extremely important and profitable discussion testified to the church's concern for the prevention and cure of a dreadful disease, and for the care of its victims.

Thus we arrive at some generalizations concerning biomedical innovations seen in the light of Orthodoxy's long-standing concern for the healing of human illness. The church is biased toward the transmission of life, its protection, and its healing. Consequently Orthodox moral judgment generally views the developing biomedical technologies positively, except where they seriously threaten the physical, spiritual, moral, personal, social, and ecclesial unity of life. This unity takes precedence in Orthodox Christian reflection as it addresses bioethical questions.

The discussion of both women's issues and bioethical concerns illustrates the developmental aspect of the Orthodox tradition. Placing these issues in a sacramental, kingdom-oriented perspective and perceiving them as part of the interconnectedness of human life (yet as only one aspect of life as a God-ward movement) gives them the proper spiritual grounding.

· 14 ·
"Trampling on Death"

William E. Phipps, scholar in religion and philosophy, begins his book *Death: Confronting the Reality* by emphasizing the rapid increase of interest in death in the past thirty years or so.

> Early in this century H. L. Mencken commented in *Smart Set*, "Go to any public library and look under 'Death: Human' in the card index, and you will be surprised to find how few books there are on the subject." That dearth of death literature has now been remedied. More books have been written in the past generation about death from psychological, biological, medical, historical, religious, and philosophical perspectives than had been written in the previous century.

Phipps also expresses our "awe-ful/awful ambivalence toward death"—we feel for it both "attraction and repulsion."[1]

On the one hand the contemplation of death is "awe-ful," and human beings seem to feel instinctively its wonder and mystery. Where the signs of life previously existed there follows a strange, silent absence, evoking a sense of awe. But concurrently we have a revulsion to death, a powerful sense of its undesirability. Death is to be resisted, to be struggled against.

It may be that the "awe-ful/awful" character of death is a paradox that cannot be overcome in human experience and thought and that—in spite of our human efforts through science, religion, philosophy, and psychology—can never be resolved. The reality of death cannot be faced with simple equanimity by human beings. Neutrality about death, whether intellectual or emotional, is not achieved without significantly dehumanizing ourselves. Stalin, commenting on the hundreds of thousands of victims of his ruthless purges, revealed such a passivity before the phenomenon of death: "A single death is a tragedy, a million deaths is a statistic."[2]

Contrast Stalin's banalization of death with a hymn from the Orthodox funeral service:

> Terror truly past compare is by the mystery of death inspired; now the soul and the body part, disjoined by resistless might, and their concord

is broken; and the bond of nature which made them live and grow as one, now by the edict of God is rent in twain. . . . [3]

Death is a reality we cannot ignore. For our own sake, for the sake of those who love us, and for the well-being of the societies in which we live, death must be probed, understood, and dealt with in spite of its complexity.

But just what is the meaning and place of death in Orthodox theology, pastoral practice, and ethics?

CONSIDERING DEATH

Throughout history, widely differing concepts of death have had prominence. Some have looked on death as the occasion of change from one kind of existence to another, others as dispersion of the person. Some have seen death as separation that calls for a unifying action of love, and others have perceived death to be a mere illusion in the face of the unity of all being. Others have understood death as a fiction, an appearance that is only a step in a long chain of being, while some traditions have seen it as the inevitable end to a finite human experience. Other approaches have sought to transform death into a new reality. Some have seen in it a vision of ultimate truths about our nature or found it to be a powerful motivator for life in this sphere of existence, paradoxically finding meaning for life in the experience and reality of death.[4]

The contemporary world offers its own perspectives on death,[5] and three are particularly significant. These I identify as death denied, death as real but not evil, and death victorious. To each of these Orthodox Christianity stands in opposition and presents a sharply different perspective.[6]

Death Denied. In spite of the reality of death which we experience all around us, our contemporary life-style tries to deny death's impact upon our thinking, acting, and functioning. This syndrome, of course, is not new. Among the ancients, Epicurus made the earliest and most classic statement: "Death means nothing to us, because that which has been broken down into atoms has no sensation and that which has no sensation is no concern of ours." This kind of thinking leads to the denial of death as an experienced reality: "This, the most horrifying of evils, means nothing to us, then, because so long as we are existent death is not present and wherever it is present we are nonexistent."[7]

The denial of death's reality is rampant in our society. Television and movie portrayals of death rob it of significance: hundreds die before our eyes on the screen, and it is nothing to us. In another context I once remarked that "today's practices—lonely hospital deaths, chemical embalming, 'double-lined metal caskets, with deluxe concrete water-resistant concrete vaults,' closed-casket funerals and other such 'distance-makers'— camouflage the tragedy and evil of death in our experience."[8]

The Orthodox Christian viewpoint presents a radical contrast to this perspective. As seen in the hymn quoted above, death is both real and tragic. In Chapter 4 we looked at the Orthodox teaching regarding the condition of separateness between ourselves and God, that is, sin, with all its potentialities for sickness. In Orthodox thought, the consequence of this sinful condition is expressed most powerfully and pervasively in death. Death is the proof of our fallenness, our lack of full humanity, the reality of our finiteness. As we shall see below, nothing in the Orthodox worldview as expressed vividly in its worship makes much sense without a powerful sense of the reality of death.

Death as Real but not Evil. There is another way by which the real impact of death, especially as an evil in itself, can be effectively denied—the way of existentialism. This philosophical perspective pervades popular conceptions of death today as influenced by contemporary psychology, and it is just as prevalent in many of the pastoral theology and psychology courses offered in theological schools and clinical pastoral programs in the United States.

By *existentialism* I mean that relatively amorphous mind-set which sees in any system or organizational expression a radical "inauthenticity." It focuses on the individual, emphasizing almost exclusively the individual's subjective assumption of responsibility for him- or herself. This is called "authentic" life. It means in practice that one has to devise one's own morality and make one's own choices, without the help of rules or principles.[9] This essentially means also that others can have no real place in "authentic life." But this method, it seems to me, is self-destructive. In my book on the theory of Orthodox Christian ethics I put it this way: "if there are no general truths, no objective existence, no ultimate reality which have meaning for human beings it means that life for each individual is totally ambiguous. At heart there is a nothingness about the human being who 'makes meaning' through his choices, but who also knows that this meaning has no meaning outside himself. His efforts to transcend himself are doomed to fail."[10]

Death plays an extremely important role in this worldview. Death, in its sharpness, reality, and finality, determines the pattern of existentialist thought. In its basic philosophical expressions, it is nearly always atheistic. Death means that life has no meaning at all. Reactions to this reality are despair and angst. One either commits suicide or struggles, in the acceptance of nothingness, to gain the "courage to be." Proponents may equate this approach with a radical acceptance of the reality and evil of death. Yet in the very process of dealing with death and dying, they are putting aside its reality and evil, denying its essential impact on human experience.

This attitude can be clearly seen in the branch of modern psychology that outlines the processes of grieving a death. The "stages" of mourning described by Elisabeth Kübler-Ross in *On Death and Dying* can certainly assist our understanding of how we grieve.[11] But this approach may also turn our focus completely from the reality and tragedy of death. This danger is signaled by Kübler-Ross's strangely titled sequel: *Death: The Final Stage of Growth.* Although the title of the final chapter, "Dying as the Last Stage of Growth," is remarkably acceptable from an Orthodox perspective, the title of the book sends a radically different message.

The concluding section of the book begins with these words: "There is no need to be afraid of death. It is not the end of the physical body that should worry us. Rather, our concern must be to *live* while we are alive. . . ." The paragraph continues in this individualistic strain, rejecting any significance of the interpersonal, social, corporate, communal dimension of human life. The only meaning for death is that it proves our personal need to affirm ourselves, to "grow, to become more of who you really are," and, strangely unexplained, "to reach out to other human beings." Subsequently, gratuitous injections of "heavenly" perspectives and assurances of the immortality of the "self or the spirit" are added, with the guidance that "You may interpret this in any way that makes you comfortable."[12] Nevertheless, they are clearly appendages having nothing to do with the living of life or the meaning of death.

I have dwelt on this perspective because it represents much that passes for thought on death today. From an Orthodox perspective, this view ultimately makes of the reality and evil of death a non-thing. Nothing is ever said about *why* one should grow, in *what direction* growth should move, or *what impact* eternal life after death would have on this life.

This view is tenable, of course, because of its pervading dualism of body and soul (or *self, personality, personhood, spirit,* or other such term indicating the "real" aspect of our existence). The body is again strangely ignored in this materialistic age. If, however, a human being is a composite of spirit and body, then minimizing the body when thinking about life and death causes great error.

It is important to note that in Orthodox theology the idea of the immortality of the soul is not centrally significant. In the biblical and patristic tradition the doctrine of the resurrection is central; it is an essential aspect of the ancient Christian "classical" understanding of the story of salvation. Humanity's creation in the image and likeness of God meant human responsibility to respond freely to the invitation to realize the fullness of human potential, which can take place only in communion with God. The breaking of that communion through sin provokes brokenness, disorientation, dissolution, corruption, and death.

Death is real, and it must be seen as evil, as an enemy, as "tyranny" over our existence. It cannot be ignored. The church teaches that death can be overcome only when God, who has been sinned against and rejected by us, initiates the potential reconciliation. God has done this through the incarnation of his son. The divine and the human (including both body and soul in their fullness) are united in a single person, Jesus Christ. His method of restoring humanity to fullness of life is teaching about it as the kingdom of God, manifesting this new life (in healings, among other things), and assuming the reality and evil of death himself and conquering it through his resurrection. Done for the whole world, this work of victory over death, sin, and evil is appropriated by human beings through baptism. For the church, and especially in the worship of the Orthodox church, the resurrection of Christ is the main feature of salvation.[13] The Antiochian theologian Theodore of Mopsuestia, born in the middle of the fourth century, sums up the view of the early church on this matter:

> The resurrection put the seal on all the wonders worked in the economy of Christ, and [it was] the most capital blow among all the righting of wrongs which he effected. By means of [the resurrection] death was destroyed, corruption dissolved, the passions [made to] disappear, mutability done away with, the urgings of sin extinguished, the power of Satan and the violence of demons was destroyed and the anguish of the law was overcome. To all this [is added] the promise of life eternal and immutable.[14]

Death Victorious. In the contrast to such faith, our age harbors a belief that death in its full magnitude is all that can be hoped for. Below, mention is made of the Orthodox ethical approaches to suicide and euthanasia. These alternatives, previously rejected, have resurfaced since the inauguration of the nuclear age. A widespread acceptance of annihilation persists in the face of the nuclear stand-off between the superpowers. Whether the predictions are of drastic environmental consequences or total destruction of the human race, the feeling pervades that we are approaching an end to life as we know it. Our ability to destroy ourselves provokes a variety of secular eschatological stances which seek somehow to overcome this assurance of the dominance of death.

At a time when hope seems to have disappeared from our consciousness, one can see the existential perspective ("live life *now!*") of Kübler-Ross proliferating in a wide range of hedonistic pursuits as disparate as the "recreational" use of drugs, the self-absorption in frenetic rock music, the scrambling after "new age" mysticisms, and the graspings after technological wonders to fend off the eventual victory of death. Let just one example, a humorous one, suffice. Phipps pokes fun at those who would achieve immortality by having their ashes rocketed into space in order to achieve an ersatz immortality:

> The latest endeavor of the multi-billion-dollar United States funeral industry has been a high-tech form of air burial. . . . For only $3,900, Celestis will compact cremains into a tiny titanium capsule, place it in the three-hundred-pound nose cone of a rocket, and blast it to kingdom come, along with 10,329 other capsules. Somewhat like the eternal orbiting of the medieval angels, this celestial cemetery will circle at nineteen hundred miles above the earth for sixty-three million years. The highly reflective surface of the spacecraft will enable relatives to watch their deceased pass overhead on clear nights. This is only the first giant leap for the ashes of humanity. . . . For those with faith in the god of technology, this final devotional tribute is appropriate![15]

This tongue-in-cheek assessment of frantic efforts to stave off an assured sense of total destruction cannot hide the despair and defeat endemic to the three views presented above. By contrast, the Christian accepts the reality of death and its evil yet maintains the conviction that death is not victorious, that in the saving work of Jesus Christ, there is victory over death.

The Orthodox expression of this conviction is not limited to words said or sung at a funeral, nor reserved for obligatory mention at the paschal season. It is the constant refrain of Orthodox worship. Every Sunday is a commemoration of the resurrection of Christ and as such a "little Easter." The vesper services of Saturday night, the services of Sunday morning, and the Divine Liturgy itself affirm each week, in a cycle of eight texts based on the eight tones of Orthodox ecclesial music, the refrain of victory over death the enemy, through Christ. Again and again the hymns proclaim this victory, as a few typical hymns from the "first tone" of the vespers illustrate:

> Rejoice, O heaven, blow the horn, ye foundations of the earth, and cry, O mountains with joy; for behold, Immanuel hath nailed our sins upon his Cross; and the Life-giver hath caused death to die, raising Adam; for he loves humankind.

Let us, though unworthy, stand by thy life-giving tomb, O Christ our Lord, and let us offer glory to thine ineffable compassion; for thou didst accept crucifixion and death, O sinless One, that thou mightest grant resurrection to the world; for thou art good and thou lovest humankind.

Let creation rejoice and the heavens have joy; and let the nations clap their hands together with gladness; for Christ our Savior did nail our sins upon his Cross; and in causing death to die, did grant us life and did raise fallen Adam and all his descendants; for he loves humankind.[16]

THE ORTHODOX WAY WITH DEATH

The Orthodox church's confidence that the Christian shares in the victory of Christ over death does not make it insensitive to the human experience of death. But the sense of victory never departs either. Before looking at contemporary Orthodox funeral practices, we need to consider briefly the undergirding beliefs about the dead.

Last Things. The doctrinal teaching of the Orthodox church holds that upon death, each person shares in a "partial judgment," a foretaste of one's eternal destiny. Though a minority view opines that there can be development or growth or change in the deceased after death, mainline teaching holds that once one has died, no further spiritual or moral progress can be made.

Nevertheless, all Orthodox authorities maintain that intercessory prayer on behalf of the deceased not only is helpful to those who remain but is in some undefined way helpful to the deceased. This middle state will remain until Christ's Second Coming, to be accompanied by the general resurrection, the Final Judgment, and the end of the world as we know it. This will be brought about by God in his time and plan, unprovoked by anything in our behavior. After the Second Coming and Judgment, the tradition holds, each person will continue to experience relatedness and communion with God (that is, the eternal kingdom of God) or, in contrast, eternal separation from God (that is, hell). Eastern Orthodoxy contains no doctrine of purgatory.

Funeral Rites. Ancient descriptions of the deaths of Christians often included the gathering of relatives and friends around the bed of the dying person. Scholars see this as part of a tradition of dealing with the dead and the dying which reaches with a "startling continuity" from antiquity to modern times.[17] In Greek village life to this day, the immediate response to a death takes two forms: laments for the deceased out of a popular tradition having roots in ancient Greece[18] and the rites of the church, which, as we shall see below, include expressions of personal loss, wonderment at death, and very personal sorrow. In the American scene, the former tradition has all but disappeared. What remains is the cycle of the church's rites regarding death and burial.

In the Orthodox tradition, as we saw in Chapter 10, the administration of Holy Communion is the usual "last rite." When the dying person is unconscious and therefore not able to receive Holy Communion, some priests will anoint the ill person, but this remains a sacrament of healing and not a death rite.

When a person dies, the parish priest is customarily called.[19] His first task is liturgical: to read the short prayer service usually referred to as the Trisaghion (the name comes from the "thrice-holy" prayers with which it begins). This may take place at the deathbed, in the hospital, or at home, with the family present or not, depending on local practice, traditions, or circumstances. The priest may then visit the bereaved family members to provide comfort and support.

In earlier times, a ritual of closing the eyes and mouth of the deceased, washing the body, anointing it with perfumed oils, wrapping it in a white shroud or in burial clothes set aside especially for this moment, and preparing it for the viewing, or *prothesis,* was performed by family members. In villages in Greece this practice has continued from Byzantine times.[20] In America, nearly all these rituals have been taken over by the funeral director, except possibly selection of the burial clothing.

In an earlier day, the deceased was "laid out" in the home, and visitors came to express condolences. The casket was open, as it is now at the funeral home. Each evening of the viewing the priest visits the funeral home at an appointed hour and reads the Trisaghion service. (It may also be read, in smaller communities, just prior to the procession to the church for the funeral service.) This is all that remains of the tradition of bearing the open casket from the home to the church for the funeral. According to one commentator on Orthodox funeral customs, the open casket indicated then and now the church's interest in conveying "the reality of death, and the wonderment created by it, which it never wished to neutralize by coverings. For the Church death is a 'teaching event' which must be left open and free to speak its eloquent and dramatic message."[21]

The content of the Orthodox funeral service is relatively fixed today, though it has developed over the centuries. In the earliest period of the church a prayer was read at the home before the procession to the house of worship. The fourth-century *Sacramentary of Serapion* contains an impressive prayer that seems to have been modified later for inclusion in the Trisaghion service and the funeral service itself.

It appears that originally psalms, Scripture readings on the resurrection, and some hymns, all attached to the Eucharist, made up the funeral service.[22] As the years went by the funeral elements expanded. The sixth-century *Ecclesiastical Hierarchy*, by Pseudo-Dionysius, describes the funeral service of that period.[23] Following the Divine Liturgy, the body is placed in the nave, close to the altar table and facing east. The service consists of psalms, hymns, Scripture readings focusing on the resurrection, and prayers by the clergy for the forgiveness of sins and for the acceptance of the deceased "in the land of the living . . . where there is neither pain, nor sorrow, nor suffering." At the end, those in attendance file by for the "final greeting." By the end of the sixth century, the present-day Orthodox funeral service "existed in outline and with its main points."[24]

This funeral service was enriched during the ninth century by a magnificent collection of eight funeral hymns written by St. John of Damascus. The set of hymns is cast as a drama in which the priest, the congregation, and the deceased are given voice. During this period variations of this service developed for use at the death of laypersons, monks, priests, and infants.[25]

Traditionally, a procession then took place from the church to the burial grounds, known as a *koimeterion* ("a place of sleep"), from which we obtain our English word *cemetery*. In the United States, all that now remains of this procession is the priest's leading the now-closed casket out of the church to the hearse and from the hearse to the burial site. The hymn usually sung, in a slow, dirgelike fashion, is the "thrice-holy" hymn, "Holy God, Holy Mighty, Holy Immortal, have mercy on us."

Because in earlier times the casket was still open, the committal service was performed at the graveside. Today, in the United States, the committal usually comes at the end of the funeral service, following the "last greeting" and the final closing of the casket. Earth and perfumed oil are placed on the body in the form of a cross, as the words "dust thou art, and to dust thou shall return" (Genesis 3:19b) and "purge me with hyssop and I shall be clean, wash me and I shall be whiter than snow" (Psalm 51:7) are repeated. At the graveside, the Trisaghion service is once again repeated.

The practice of gathering the mourners for a memorial meal immediately after the funeral grew out of the long-standing tradition of doing charity in the name of the deceased.[26] It has obvious psychological value for the living as well. Were it not for these meals, the family of the deceased would have, as they went to the privacy of their homes, the fresh memory of the open grave. With the meal another experience is placed between that event and the inevitable moment of loneliness, and it is a social event, in which the mourning family is reincorporated after a fashion into the larger community. The Greek Orthodox refer to these meals as "forgiveness meals," implying both the prayers for the forgiveness of the sins of the deceased as well as the putting to an end of differences and quarrels in the community in which the deceased may have been involved.

But the end of the funeral rites does not end the mourning period. Marked by a series of memorial services, this lasts for a year. Though ancient traditions call for services to be conducted on the third, the ninth, and the fortieth day from the death, followed by the six-month and anniversary services, it is more common in the U.S. for the first memorial service to be conducted on the fortieth day. This service consists of some hymns from the funeral and the Trisaghion services, together with the presentation of a tray of sweetened, boiled wheat. The wheat reflects the words of Jesus regarding death and resurrection: "unless a grain of wheat falls into the earth and dies, it remains alone; but if it dies it bears much fruit" (John 12:24). The memorial service, like the funeral service, ends with the repetition of a haunting hymn that calls for "eternal memory" for the deceased. Subsequently, the name of the deceased will be included in lists of the dead for commemoration at the Divine Liturgy and on special "Saturdays of Souls" at different times throughout the church year.

Liturgical Messages. The cycle of services just described carries with it a wide range of messages—that death is real, evil, and painful, that it challenges life's ordinary values and can be devastating if faced without faith, that it calls us to repentance, that it is overcome by Christ's victory over death, and that through faith death can even become a manifestation of the kingdom of God. The service itself, with its dialogic character, can allow for final communication with the deceased, a final farewell, and an emotional release. The presence of the open casket and the language of mourning and grief can contribute to the mourners' acceptance of the death of the loved one.

Several authors have analyzed the service from their own perspectives. Paul J. Fedwick lists several theological ideas emphasized in the service, among them the theme of separation—of the soul from the body, of the deceased from the world, from relatives, from habits of conduct. He notes that this separation is also presented as "translation from corruption to eschatological eternity" in repose, rest, and "falling asleep." Here the reality of deterioration and destruction is not hidden. A third theological motif is that death itself is the "beginning of liberation": death is now understood as vanquished, as an object of "thanksgiving," since in Christ it is entry into the kingdom. Lamentation and rejoicing are intertwined in the loss of the loved one and the hope of the resurrection.[27]

Boris Bobrinskoy, an Orthodox priest serving in France, emphasizes the communal aspect of the funeral rites, or the "sacrament of death," as he calls it:

> Within the community of the Church, the death of any member of the Body of Christ is more than an event that marks the term of an individual human life. It becomes as well an event in and for the ecclesial community as a whole. Through the liturgical and spiritual celebration of death, the Church aligns itself with both the deceased and its living members. And it does so in the name of God, within the mystery of Christ's own journey through death and into resurrection . . . and thereby death acquires meaning as a sign of a "coming": not of Godot, but of God.[28]

In *The Mystery of Death*, the distinguished theologian Nicholas Vasiliades speaks of the spiritual impact of the funeral service on the family and the mourners. A funeral is a "wonderful opportunity" to understand both the sorrowful event of death and its meaning for those who remain:

> When we enter deeply into the profound thoughts expressed in the funeral service, our soul is humbled, softened. It prays deeply for the forgiveness and rest of the person who has gone over to the life beyond the grave. But we who continue in this life are brought to the decision to live the balance of our lives in repentance in a life style which is pleasing to God and Christ.[29]

The theme of the educative influence of the Orthodox funeral service is developed extensively, however, by Frank Marangos, a priest of the Greek Orthodox Archdiocese of North and South America. In "Shared Christian Praxis: Approaching the Orthodox Funeral Service," Marangos relates the dynamic of the funeral service to the process of growth in God-likeness for those who participate in the service. "At all major points," he notes, "the service attempts to thrust individual participants and the entire community beyond their present conduct, understanding, feeling, desires and relationships."[30] Besides provoking "critical reflection," the service educates through its dialogic hymnody and prayers, the story of salvation it tells in various ways, and its vision of the kingdom as a "homeland" and a place of rest. He sums up the meaning of the Orthodox funeral service as a lesson in discipleship.

Finally, an extensive treatment of the pastoral and psychological content of the service is presented by Philotheos Faros, an Orthodox priest and a professional pastoral psychologist.[31] For Faros, the funeral is a pastoral occasion for the expression of grief. He deals extensively with the negative consequences of denying death and shows how the realistic patterns in the Orthodox funeral service allow for a full acceptance of its reality and the opportunity for a complete expression of mourning.[32] Faros holds that the service, in allowing a form of direct conversation *with* the deceased and not merely about him, permits formerly unsaid things to be said. From the perspective of the psychology of mourning, this opportunity to confess wrongs and seek forgiveness is significant. The possibility of touching the body of the deceased in the open casket and the offering of parting greetings in the church provide for a "climate of therapeutic grief."[33] Faros also outlines the psychology of the Orthodox funeral, which includes (1) the love of God as a counterpoint to the feeling of being orphaned, (2) an assessment of life and the tragedy of death, (3) a realistic evaluation of the loss of a life, and the sense of the insecurity of this life, (4) the sorrow for death and the means to grieve, (5) the death and resurrection of Christ as an anchor of hope for our human existence, and (6) the formalized "leave-taking" in the last greeting in the church.[34]

Making this whole complex of realities possible, and giving it cohesion, balance, and direction, of course, is the shared belief and experience of the resurrection of Christ. At Easter, the dismissal hymn sums up the whole approach of the Orthodox church to death:

> Christ is risen from the dead!
> By His death,
> trampling on Death,
> And to those in the tombs,
> He gives life.

A Brief Word on Ethics and Death. The funeral service emphasizes the reality of death and its evil and accepts death as a human reality, yet it also affirms victory over death through the sharing in the resurrection of Jesus Christ. Related to these stances is the Orthodox ethical tradition of affirming life and accepting bioethical positions that support that perspective.[35] As we saw in the preceding chapter, ethical decisions about life are rooted in the biblical, patristic, doctrinal, canonical, spiritual, and liturgical tradition of the church. It is no less the case as the Orthodox church addresses the moral questions related to death.

On Abortion. The teaching of the Orthodox church has consistently opposed abortion, because it considers it a form of murder. Those who confess to the sin may be forgiven through the sacrament of holy confession, though the father confessor has wide discretion in the matter. Little flexibility exists in principle, with the main exception in ethical teaching being the saving of the threatened life of the mother. This position is documented in some of the earliest patristic material, such as the second-century *Didache of the Twelve Apostles,* and has been consistently repeated in numerous pronouncements to this very day.[36]

On Euthanasia. On the other end of the spectrum, the Orthodox tradition has always strongly opposed active promotion of euthanasia.[37] The active taking of another's life is seen as a special case of murder and condemned as such. However, the development of medical technologies that permit the continued functioning of the body beyond the generally accepted criteria related to "brain death" has complicated the issue and provoked discussion. In contemporary Orthodox thinking, there is place for "allowing" a person to die when it is clear that efforts at maintaining life are futile. This is based on a long-standing tradition predating the rise of modern medicine, expressed in an ancient service in the main prayer book of the church, the Service at the Tearing Away of the Soul. It was written to address cases when dying was particularly difficult and long-lasting. Of course, the thrust of the service was to ask God to "take" the dying person, the most that human beings could do in such circumstances. The service has never been perceived as an act of euthanasia.

On Martyrdom. The church's hierarchy of values becomes clear in its approach to the issue of voluntary and involuntary martyrdom. From the earliest of times, the church has rejected the provocation of martyrdom by Christians: no one is to put his or her life, which is valued highly by the church, at unnecessary risk. However, when one is challenged to deny faith in Christ, resistance to apostasy may mean acceptance of martyrdom.

On Autopsy. Some Orthodox believers, having a strong sense of the integrity of the body, resist autopsies, but this is far from being a universal practice. The church makes no formal objection to these procedures, provided that the bodily remains of the deceased are respected and returned intact for burial. Again, the issue is respect for the wholeness of the physical and spiritual dimensions of life.

On the Donation of Organs. No clear and unambiguous teaching regarding the donation of organs is fully accepted in the Orthodox church. Nevertheless, the recent encyclical letter from the archbishop of Athens announcing his personal decision to donate certain of his organs after death has given impetus to the practice. A stipulation understood by Orthodoxy is that the donor's body be buried properly and accorded full respect. The donation of organs from the living has been debated among the Orthodox, as among other groups, but there has been no widespread objection. Qualified support has been given, following the reasoning that the motive of love and charity for the patient who has need of an organ justifies such donations. Nevertheless, the cautions in the general ethical literature on the subject need to be respected as well. For example, the Orthodox would hold that there is no moral law *demanding* organ donations, that the giving of an organ should be a free act of love which does not put one's own life in jeopardy, and that close relatives who opt not to donate organs should be given a measure of protection from criticism. Nevertheless, the church encourages those who donate organs to do so out of a philanthropic motive.

The donation of bodies to medical schools, though not disapproved formally, is not often encouraged. The perception brought from Europe is that the bodies of such persons are not treated with due respect in those circumstances. Nevertheless, where cadavers receive appropriate attention and arrangements are made for rites of burial after their scientific educational use, there are no fundamental ethical objections; it is thought practically and prudentially better for students to learn about organs and medical procedures with cadavers than with living human beings. The issues, rather, are practical and pastoral. How can pastoral attention to the mourning process of the relatives be given when almost immediate possession of the body of the deceased is required by the medical school? When are the traditional funeral rites to be conducted? Though these need not be insurmountable problems, they have not been worked out yet by the Orthodox in a coherent way.

Immediately after the death, a brief service could perhaps gather the family and friends, with a memorial service at the church following a few days later. This would allow the mourning process to begin. A funeral/burial service could follow a year or so later when the body was returned to the family. Medical schools allowing that kind of treatment of the body (keeping the body parts together and returning the body to the family for burial) will find greater support among the Orthodox for the donation of bodies to science.

On Cremation. The Orthodox church, with its strong doctrine of the resurrection of the body, generally has not practiced cremation and at present in the U.S. will not conduct funeral services for people planning to have their remains cremated. Some Orthodox jurisdictions, however, may permit the chanting of the Trisaghion service for these persons.

Throughout the Orthodox approach to death we see a supreme confidence that Jesus Christ himself died for the salvation of humanity and that through his resurrection, he is victor over death. Orthodox Christianity is unintelligible without that central affirmation. It celebrates Jesus as the "beginning, the first-born from the dead" (Colossians 1:18), for "in fact, Christ has been raised from the dead, the first fruits of those who have fallen asleep" (1 Corinthians 15:20). Consequently, the Orthodox have adopted as their own the age-old affirmation of triumph over death, first articulated in the thirteenth chapter of the Old Testament prophet Hosea, and reiterated by St. Paul in the fifteenth chapter of his first letter to the Christians of Corinth. Immersed in resurrection faith, the Orthodox church leads its people—after all else has been said and done in regard to death—to a confidence that the power of death has been subdued, that fear and anxiety regarding death have been overcome, and that, in essence, death has been destroyed. With Hosea and Paul the Orthodox church challenges and proclaims: " 'O death, where is thy victory? / O death, where is thy sting?' . . . thanks be to God, who gives us the victory through our Lord Jesus Christ."

Notes

Chapter 1/ Tradition and History

1. As is the case with any survey, much must be left out, and much of what is said may provoke further interest. For readers interested in further study of Orthodox Christianity several sources are recommended. Probably the best introduction in English is Timothy Ware's *Orthodox Church* (Baltimore: Penguin Books, most recent edition). Useful for topical references is Nicon D. Patrinacos's *Dictionary of Greek Orthodoxy* (New York: Greek Orthodox Archdiocese, 1984). For short essays on various aspects of the Orthodox faith tradition, see Fotios K. Litsas, *A Companion to the Greek Orthodox Church* (New York: Greek Orthodox Archdiocese Department of Communications, 1984). A more detailed historical description of Eastern Orthodoxy is given in John Meyendorff, *The Orthodox Church: Its Past and Its Role in the World Today* (Crestwood, N.Y.: St. Vladimir's Seminary Press, 1981), and Alexander Schmemann, *The Historical Road of Eastern Orthodoxy* (Crestwood, N.Y.: St. Vladimir's Seminary Press, 1977). For a biblically centered approach to Orthodox spirituality, see the two volumes of Gerasimos Papadopoulos, *Orthodoxy: Faith and Life: Christ in the Gospels* and *Orthodoxy: Faith and Life: Christ in the Life of the Church* (Brookline, Mass.: Holy Cross Orthodox Press, 1980, 1981). For a popular yet serious treatment of Greek Orthodoxy, see Demetrios J. Constantelos, *Understanding the Greek Orthodox Church* (New York: Seabury Press, Harper and Row, 1982). For very brief topical treatments of questions on Eastern Orthodoxy, see Stanley S. Harakas, *The Orthodox Church: 455 Questions and Answers* (Minneapolis: Light and Life, 1987).

2. In the sixteenth century these Orthodox Christians and their clergy were absorbed into communion with Rome, even though they retained their Eastern Christian beliefs and practices (Union of Brest-Litovsk, 1595). The Orthodox called them Uniates, while the West preferred the term Eastern-rite Catholics. In the U.S. Ukrainian and Romanian Uniate groups returned to the Orthodox church. There are Maronite, Melchite, Ruthenian, Carpathian, and other such bodies in the U.S. today. Jurisdictionally they are under the pope of Rome, and many were slowly being latinized until Vatican II, when the new policy encouraged the maintenance and development of their Eastern characteristics.

3. "Today, in addition to the four ancient Patriarchates of the East, there are four modern patriarchates, four autocephalous [self-governing] churches, and three autonomous [partially dependent] churches, as determined by the Ecumenical Pa-

triarchate of Constantinople. Many of these churches are national or cultural in character, such as the churches of Greece, Russia, Romania, Yugoslavia (Serbia), and Finland." Stanley Samuel Harakas, "The Eastern Orthodox Tradition," in *Caring and Curing: Health and Medicine in the Western Religious Traditions*, ed. Ronald L. Numbers and Darrel W. Amundsen (New York: Macmillan, 1986), p. 147.

Chapter 2/ Faith, Ethos, and Experience

1. Excellent treatments of the history of Orthodox doctrinal development can be found in Jaroslav Pelikan's *Spirit of Eastern Christendom (600–1700)*, vol. 2 of *The Christian Tradition: A History of the Development of Doctrine* (Chicago: University of Chicago Press, 1974), and in John Meyendorff's *Byzantine Theology: Historical Trends and Doctrinal Themes* (New York: Fordham University Press, 1974). A systematic approach to Orthodox doctrine can be found in Vladimir Lossky's *Mystical Theology of the Eastern Church* (London: James Clarke, 1973).

2. For more detail about the place of the Orthodox clergy in the life of the Orthodox community, see Stanley S. Harakas, "An Orthodox Perspective," chap. 10 in *Ministry in America: A Report and Analysis, Based on an In-Depth Survey of 47 Denominations in the United States and Canada, with Interpretation by 18 Experts*, ed. David S. Schuller et al. (New York: Harper and Row, 1980).

3. For a brief appraisal of the Greek Orthodox in America, see Demetrios J. Constantelos, *Understanding the Greek Orthodox Church: Its Faith, History and Practice* (New York: Seabury Press, 1982), chap. 5. An important work on Greek Orthodoxy in the U.S. is George Papaioannou's *Odyssey of Hellenism in America* (Thessalonica: Patriarchal Institute for Patristic Studies, 1985). A sociological approach is found in Charles C. Moskos, Jr., *Greek Americans: Struggle and Success* (Englewood Cliffs, N.J.: Prentice-Hall, 1980).

4. Leonidas Contos gives a pessimistic view of this issue in *2001: The Church in Crisis* (Brookline, Mass.: Holy Cross Orthodox Press, 1982).

5. A record of this outreach is to be found in Stanley S. Harakas, *Let Mercy Abound: Social Concern in the Greek Orthodox Church* (Brookline, Mass.: Holy Cross Orthodox Press, 1983).

Chapter 3/ A Wholistic Perspective

1. For example, regarding the Bible, see *Theological Dictionary of the New Testament*, ed. Gerhard Kittel and Gerhard Friedrich, trans. Geoffrey W. Bromily (Grand Rapids: Wm. B. Eerdmans, 1971), 7:965–1024.

2. John 4:42, 1 John 4:14. Unless otherwise noted, references throughout are to the Revised Standard Version.

3. Gustaf Aulén, *Christus Victor: An Historical Study of the Three Main Types of the Idea of the Atonement*, trans. A. G. Hebert (London: S.P.C.K., 1965), pp. 158–59.

4. Quoted from *Against Heresies* 5.21.3 in Aulén, *Christus Victor*, p. 34.

5. Ibid., p. 159.

6. *The Festal Menaion*, trans. Mother Mary and Archimandrite Kallistos Ware (London: Faber and Faber, 1977), p. 134.

7. Nikos A. Matsoukas, *Dogmatic and Symbolic Theology 2: Exposition of the Orthodox Faith Contrasted with Western Christianity* (in Greek) (Thessalonica: P. Pournaras Publications, 1985), p. 525. The passage continues: "It is a fact that scholastic theology is poor in therapeutic terminology and very rich in legal terminology. This constitutes a factor which differentiates Western theology from Orthodox theology." All translations are my own unless noted otherwise.

8. Ibid., p. 526.

9. St. Basil, "To Eustathius the Physician," Letter 181, *The Nicene and Post-Nicene Fathers*, 2d ser. (Grand Rapids, Mich.: Wm. B. Eerdmans, 1952–57), 8: 228–29.

10. I am using here the translation from the Library of Christian Classics series. Vol. 4, *Cyril of Jerusalem and Nemesius of Emesa*, ed. William Telfer (Philadelphia: Westminster Press, 1955), pp. 19–192. The topics relating to the body are covered in secs. 22–30, pp. 110–15. Cyril speaks once again about the body when he considers the issue of the resurrection of the body, in Lecture 18, pp. 178–85. This volume is hereafter cited as Telfer.

11. Irenaeus, another early writer (130–200 C.E.) described views like these among the heretical Carpocratians and the Nicolaitans in his *Against Heresies* 1. 25–26.

12. 1 Timothy 4:1–5; Revelation 2:4, 15.

13. Cyril of Jerusalem, *Catecheses*, Lecture 4, in Telfer, p. 111.

14. *Triads in Defense of the Holy Hesychasts* 1.2.1, in *Gregory Palamas: The Triads*, ed. John Meyendorff, trans. Nicholas Gendle (New York: Paulist Press, 1983), p. 41.

15. Cyril of Jerusalem, *Catecheses*, Lecture 4, in Telfer, p. 111.

16. Ibid., p. 112.

17. Ibid., p. 113.

18. St. Paul's teaching is normative for Orthodox Christianity: "Now if Christ is preached as raised from the dead, how can some of you say that there is no resurrection of the dead? But if there is no resurrection of the dead, then Christ has not been raised; if Christ has not been raised, then our preaching is in vain and your faith is in vain . . . and you are still in your sins. . . . If for this life only we have hoped in Christ, we are of all men most to be pitied" (1 Corinthians 15:12–14, 17b, 19).

19. Cyril of Jerusalem, *Catecheses*, Lecture 4, in Telfer, p. 184.

20. Ibid., pp. 184–85.

21. See, for example, St. Maximus the Confessor, "Four Hundred Texts on Love." *The Philokalia*, trans. G. E. H. Palmer, Philip Sherrard, and Kallistos Ware, 3 vols. to date (London: Faber and Faber, 1979–), 2:91. (The original Greek edition now in print consists of five volumes.)

22. Margaret R. Miles, *Historical Foundations for a New Asceticism* (Philadelphia: Westminster Press, 1981), pp. 139–40.

23. *The Praktikos*, trans. John E. Bamberger (Kalamazoo, Mich.: Cistercian Publications, 1970), p. 61.

Chapter 4/ Illness

1. "Fourth Century of Various Texts," no. 78. *Philokalia* 2:257. (The century, a collection of 100 short reflections on a common topic, is a literary form used frequently in the *Philokalia*.)
2. "On the Spiritual Law," no. 2. *Philokalia* 1:110.
3. "On Spiritual Knowledge and Discrimination," no. 78. *Philokalia* 1:280 (translation here slightly revised).
4. "Various Texts on Theology, the Divine Economy, and Virtue and Vice," no. 47. *Philokalia* 1:248.
5. *Philokalia* 3:343.
6. "A Treasury of Divine Knowledge," bk. 1, "God's Universal and Particular Gifts." *Philokalia* 3:172.
7. "Gnomic Anthology," 1.10. *Philokalia* 3:35.
8. "On Spiritual Knowledge and Discrimination," no. 94. *Philokalia* 1:290.
9. "Outline Teaching on Asceticism and Stillness in the Solitary Life." *Philokalia* 1:36.
10. "For the Encouragement of the Monks in India Who Had Written to Him," no. 12. *Philokalia* 1:301.
11. "On the Eight Vices." *Philokalia* 1:74.
12. "On Spiritual Knowledge and Discrimination," no. 53. *Philokalia* 1:267–68.
13. For a fuller treatment, see Stanley S. Harakas, *Toward Transfigured Life: Toward a Theoria of Orthodox Christian Ethics* (Minneapolis: Light and Life, 1983), chap. 4.
14. "Practical Chapters," 1st century, no. 88. *Philokalia* (Greek ed.), 3:294.
15. "Second Century on Love," nos. 76, 78. *Philokalia* 2:78.
16. "Fourth Century on Love," no. 66. *Philokalia* 2:108.

Chapter 5/ Suffering

1. Alexander F. C. Webster, "Typologies for an Orthodox Pastoral Theology of Physical Suffering," *Diakonia* 15, no. 2 (1980): 134.
2. *An Orthodox Prayer Book*, ed. N. M. Vaporis, trans. John von Holzhausen and Michael Gelsinger (Brookline, Mass.: Holy Cross Orthodox Press, 1977), p. 100.
3. *Service Book of the Holy Orthodox-Catholic Apostolic Church*, trans. Isabel Florence Hapgood, 6th ed. (Englewood, N.J.: Antiochian Orthodox Christian Archdiocese of North America, 1983), pp. 11–12. The translation is here revised to alter archaic spelling and language.
4. Demetrios J. Constantelos, *Byzantine Philanthropy and Social Welfare* (New Brunswick, N.J.: Rutgers University Press, 1968). A short description of Byzantine philanthropic activity in the reign of a single Byzantine emperor is described in Constantelos's article "Philanthropy in the Age of Justinian," *Greek Orthodox Theological Review* 6, no. 2 (1960–61): 206–26.

5. St. John Chrysostom, "Homilies on the Epistle to the Hebrews," *Nicene and Post-Nicene Fathers* 14:384.

6. Ibid.

7. "Homilies on the Epistles of Paul to the Corinthians," Homily 12, 4. *Nicene and Post-Nicene Fathers* 12:339.

8. "Homilies on Hebrews," Homily 28, 6. *Nicene and Post-Nicene Fathers* 14:494.

9. Ibid., 7, p. 494.

10. Ibid., 8, p. 495.

11. "The Suffering and Death of Children," *Eastern Churches Review* 8, no. 2 (1976): 107–12.

12. "On Providence," secs. 19, 33. Quoted in James Walsh and P. J. Walsh, *Divine Providence and Human Suffering* (Wilmington, Del.: Michael Glazier, 1985), p. 131.

13. See, for example, canons 1–9 of the regional Synod of Ancyra (314 C.E.). The epitome of the ninth canon of St. Peter the Martyr, archbishop of Alexandria, reads: "they who provoked the magistrates to persecute themselves and others are to be blamed. . . . " *Ancient Epitome of the Sacred Canons of the Eastern Orthodox Church,* ed. George Mastrantonis (St. Louis: OLOGOS, n.d.).

14. "Homilies on Hebrews," Homily 5, 7. *Nicene and Post-Nicene Fathers* 14:392.

15. "Homilies on the Second Epistle of St. Paul the Apostle to Timothy," Homily 8, 5.14. *Nicene and Post-Nicene Fathers* 13:507.

16. "Homilies on the Statues," 1.14. *Nicene and Post-Nicene Fathers* 9:336.

17. "A Treasury of Divine Knowledge." *Philokalia* 3:77–78.

18. Just one example is Alexander Webster's "Exemplary Kenotic Holiness of Prince Myshkin in Dostoyevsky's *The Idiot," St. Vladimir's Theological Quarterly* 28, no. 3 (1984):189–216, where further references to the literary analysis of kenoticism can be found.

19. Anita and Peter Deyneka, Jr., *Christianity Today,* 16 July 1982, p. 20.

Chapter 6/ Human Dignity in Caring and Curing

1. Ecclesiasticus is also known by the names "The Wisdom of Jesus the Son of Sirach," "Ben Sira," or simply "Sirach." On its dating by scholars, see *The Oxford Dictionary of the Christian Church,* ed. F. L. Cross (London: Oxford University Press, 1963), s.v. "Ecclesiasticus."

2. Ecclesiasticus 38:9–15. *The Septuagint Version of the Old Testament and Apocrypha* (New York: Samuel Bagster and Sons, n.d.). "As not being," the last phrase of verse 11, lacks clarity in this translation, even though it is accurately translated from the Greek *os me hyparchon.* Here I have substituted the Revised Standard Version's translation of the Hebrew "as much as you can afford," as making better sense.

3. "Peri tis Anthropou Kataskeves" (On the Construction of Man), 1.6. *Patrologia Graeca,* ed. J. P. Migne, 162 vols. (Paris, 1857–66), 30:16 (hereafter cited as *PG*).

4. *Exposition of the Orthodox Faith* 2:12. *Nicene and Post-Nicene Fathers*, 2d ser., 9:31 (in the second part of the volume).

5. *Philokalia* 1:361.

6. "Eis to Poiesomen Anthropon" (On the Words 'Let Us Create Man'), 1. *PG* 44:273.

7. "Peri tis Anthropou Kataskeves," 1.20. *PG* 30:29.

8. Constantelos, *Byzantine Philanthropy*, chaps. 1–3.

9. Quoted in Eusebius, *Church History* 7.23.7–8, 10. *Nicene and Post-Nicene Fathers*, 2d ser., 1:307.

10. Constantelos, *Byzantine Philanthropy*.

11. David Allen and Victoria S. Allen, *Ethical Issues in Mental Retardation* (Nashville: Abingdon, 1979), p. 35.

12. Ibid., p. 10.

13. *Euchologion to Mega* (The Great Book of Prayers), ed. Spyridon Zervos (Athens: Aster Publishing House, 1970), pp. 151–52, 156.

14. Ibid.

15. Aristotle Chr. Eutychiades and Spyros G. Marketos, "Medical Psychology and Mental Health in Accordance to the Greek Medical Texts from 1453 to the Middle of the 19th Century" (in Greek), *Theologia* 57, no. 1 (1986): 174–78. See also Blair Justice, *Who Gets Sick: Thinking and Health* (Houston: Peak Press, 1987).

16. A recent expression of a rejection of modern psychological therapies is Michael Nedelsky's "Contemporary Clinical Psychology: An Orthodox Perspective," *Orthodox Life* 35, nos. 4–5 (1985): 34–48.

17. Examples of this approach are some of the writings of Philotheos Faros: "Mental Patients and Verbal Communication of the Religious Message," *Theologia* 42 (1971): 602–6; *Mourning: An Orthodox, Popular and Psychological Assessment* (in Greek), Psychology-Pastoral Theology series, no. 2. (Athens: Akritas Publications, 1981). Also using this approach in the U.S. is Joseph Allen of the Antiochian Archdiocese and St. Vladimir's Orthodox Seminary, and to some extent John Chirban, Hellenic College, Brookline, Massachusetts.

18. A few representative titles: *The Crisis of Puberty, Health, Illness and the Psyche of Youth, Psychoanalysis and the Synthesis of Existence, Woman and Her Psychology, The Psychological Examination of the Child, Topics of Contemporary Psychology, The Psychological Maturity of Human Beings*, and *Abnormal and Mal-Adjusted Children*.

19. "The Suffering and Death of Children," pp. 109–10.

Chapter 7/ Doctors, Priests, and Rational Medicine

1. *De praescriptione haereticorum* 7.3. *The Ante-Nicene Fathers* (Grand Rapids, Mich.: Wm. B. Eerdmans, 1950–51), 3:246.

2. *Against Heresies*, vol. 1 of *Ante-Nicene Fathers* (1867; reprint, Grand Rapids, Mich.: Wm. B. Eerdmans, 1975).

3. *The Oxford Dictionary of the Christian Church*, ed. F. L. Cross (London: Oxford University Press, 1963), s.v. "Cappadocian Fathers."

4. See Mary Emily Keenan's "Gregory of Nazianzus and Early Byzantine Medicine," *Bulletin of the History of Medicine* 9 (1941): 8–30, and "St. Gregory of Nyssa and the Medical Profession," *Bulletin of the History of Medicine* 15 (1944): 150–61.

5. Darrel W. Amundsen, "Medicine and Faith in Early Christianity," *Bulletin of the History of Medicine* 56 (1982): 341.

6. For a contemporary Orthodox effort to focus on the synthetic, rather than the discontinuous, see *Orthodox Synthesis: The Unity of Theological Thought*, ed. Joseph J. Allen (Crestwood, N.Y.: St. Vladimir's Seminary Press, 1981).

7. For a wide range of texts of the Byzantine era, see Deno John Geanakoplos, *Byzantium: Church, Society, and Civilization Seen through Contemporary Eyes* (Chicago: University of Chicago Press, 1984). For some texts of Byzantine writers on social issues, see *Social and Political Thought in Byzantium: From Justinian I to the Last Palaeologus*, trans. Ernest Barker (Oxford: Clarendon Press, 1957). For patristic writings of both East and West, see *The Early Church and the State*, ed. Agnes Cunningham (Philadelphia: Fortress Press, 1982). See also Steven Runciman, *The Orthodox Church and the Secular State* (Oxford: Oxford University Press, 1971). For a contemporary assessment, see Aristeides Papadakis, "The Historical Tradition of Church-State Relations under Orthodoxy," in *Eastern Christianity and Politics in the Twentieth Century*, ed. Pedro Ramet (Durham, N.C.: Duke University Press, 1988), chap. 3.

8. John Scarborough, ed., *Symposium on Byzantine Medicine, Dumbarton Oaks Papers 38* (Washington, D.C.: Dumbarton Oaks Research Library and Collection, 1985), p. ix.

9. Arnold J. Toynbee, *A Study of History*, abr. D. C. Somervell (New York: Oxford University Press, 1953), p. 82.

10. Scarborough, *Byzantine Medicine*, pp. x, xi.

11. See John Duffy, "Byzantine Medicine in the Sixth and Seventh Centuries: Aspects of Teaching and Practice," in *Byzantine Medicine*, ed. Scarborough, 21–27.

12. Aristotle Chr. Eutychiades, *The Practice of Byzantine Medical Science and Its Social Application According to Related Regulations* (in Greek) (Athens: Gregory K. Parisianos, 1983). See also Demetrios J. Constantelos, "The Interface of Medicine and Religion in the Greek and the Christian Greek Orthodox Tradition," *Greek Orthodox Theological Review* 33, no. 1 (1988): 1–17.

13. *The Instructor* 1.2. *Ante-Nicene Fathers* 1:210.

14. "Homilies on the Statues," Homily 5, 19. *Nicene and Post-Nicene Fathers*, 1st ser. 9:378.

15. Timothy S. Miller, *The Birth of the Hospital in the Byzantine Empire* (Baltimore: Johns Hopkins University Press, 1985).

16. Ibid., pp. 4, 5–6.

17. Ibid., p. 4 (my emphasis).

18. Ibid., p. 61. For hospitals and health services in later Byzantium (1204–1453), see Demetrios J. Constantelos, *Poverty, Society and Philanthropy in the Late Medieval Greek World* (New York, 1989), chap. 9.

19. For more information on the Pantokrator Hospital, see Miller, *Birth of the Hospital*, chap. 2. See also Constantelos, *Byzantine Philanthropy*, chap. 11, and Timothy S. Miller, "Byzantine Hospitals," in *Byzantine Medicine*, ed. Scarborough, pp. 53–64.

20. Franz Dorbeck, "Origin of Medicine in Russia," *Medical Life* 30 (1923): 223–33; Nancy Mandelker Frieden, *Russian Physicians in an Era of Reform and Revolution (1856–1905)* (Princeton, N.J.: Princeton University Press, 1981).

21. Steven Runciman, *The Great Church in Captivity: A Study of the Patriarchate of Constantinople from the Eve of the Turkish Conquest to the Greek War of Independence* (Cambridge: Cambridge University Press, 1968), p. 213.

22. Timothy Ware, *Eustratios Argenti: A Study of the Greek Church under Turkish Rule* (Oxford: Oxford University Press, 1964), pp. 45–47.

23. In *La Théologie dans L'Eglise et dans le Monde* (Geneva: Editions du Centre Orthodoxe du Patriarchat Oecouménique, 1984), pp. 203–25.

24. I. Alexiou et al., *What Did Christianity Contribute?* vol. 3 of *Social Service during the 'Tourkokratia'* (in Greek) (Athens: Tenos Publications, 1980).

25. The comments that follow were drawn from a questionnaire circulated among Orthodox physicians, laity, and clergy regarding attitudes toward health and medicine and the Orthodox Christian faith. Here only written comments made by physicians are quoted.

26. The papers presented at the symposium appear in *Thalassemia: An Interdisciplinary Approach*, ed. John T. Chirban (Lanham, Md: University Press of America, 1986).

27. *Constitution of the Orthodox Christian Association of Medicine, Psychology and Religion*, Article II, c. Plans for the organization began under the direction of John Chirban, on the psychology faculty at Hellenic College.

28. "God in the Sphere of the Natural Sciences Today" (in Greek), in *Spiritual Gift: A Festschrift on the 50th Anniversary of Scholarly Activity and the 40th Anniversary of the Professorship and Ecclesial Activity of Gerasimos J. Konidaris* (Athens: Faculty of the Theological School of the Universary of Athens, 1981), pp. 516–17.

Chapter 8/ Spiritual Healing: The Saints

1. Amundsen, "Medicine and Faith," pp. 348–49.

2. Quoted by Phaedon Koukoules, *Byzantine Life and Society* (in Greek), 6 vols. (Athens, 1948–55), 6:11.

3. Adolf Harnack, *Medical Practice from Earliest Church History* (in German) (Leipzig, 1892); Demetrios J. Constantelos, "Physician-Priests in the Medieval Greek Church," *Greek Orthodox Theological Review* 14, no. 3 (1969): 141–53. Constantelos, "Clerics and Secular Professions in the Byzantine Church," *Byzantina* 13, no. 1 (1985): 373–90.

4. Constantelos, "Clerics and Secular Professions," p. 385.

5. See Constantelos, "Interface of Medicine and Religion," pp. 9–10.

6. William J. Lederer, *I, Giorgios* (New York: W. W. Norton, 1984), p. 28.

7. These are mentioned in many liturgical editions. A current example is *Hieratikon: Ai Theiai Leitoyrgiai* (Priest's Service Book: The Divine Liturgies) (Athens: Apostolike Diakonia, 1981), p. 67.

8. George D. Metallenos, *Threskevtike kai Ethike Engyklopaideia*, s.v. "Panteleimon." The translation is from the unpublished *Menaion* for July from St. Vladimir's Orthodox Seminary.

9. Robert Browning, "The 'Low Level' Saint's Life in the Early Byzantine World," in *The Byzantine Saint*, University of Birmingham Fourteenth Spring Symposium of Byzantine Studies, ed. Sergei Hackel, studies supplementary to *Sobornost* 5 (London: Fellowship of St. Albans and St. Sergius, 1981), pp. 122–23.

10. Peregrine Horden, "Saints and Doctors in the Early Byzantine Empire: The Case of Theodore of Sykeon," *The Church and Healing*, ed. W. J. Sheils, 1–14 (Oxford: Basil Blackwell, 1982), p. 13.

11. Ibid., p. 1.

12. According to Nicholas Gendle, "the tokens (*eulogiai*) given by the holy man to visitors may take the form of an *ampulla* or a medal (or just a fragment of clothing) that has been in physical contact with him." "The Role of the Byzantine Saint in the Development of the Icon Cult," in *Byzantine Saint*, ed. Hackel, p. 183. For similar miracles in later Byzantium see Alice-Mary M. Talbot, *Faith Healing in Late Byzantium* (Brookline, Mass.: Hellenic College Press, 1983); Constantelos, "Interface of Medicine and Religion," pp. 10–12.

13. Gary Vikan, "Art, Medicine and Magic in Early Byzantium," in *Byzantine Medicine*, ed. Scarborough, pp. 65–86; Susan Ashbrook Harvey, "Physicians and Ascetics in John of Ephesus: An Expedient Alliance," ibid., pp. 87–94; Harry J. Magoulias, "The Lives of the Saints as Sources of Data for the History of Byzantine Medicine in the Sixth and Seventh Centuries," *Byzantinische Zeitschrift* 57 (1964): 127–50.

14. Ihor Ševčenko and Nancy Patterson Ševčenko, *The Life of Saint Nicholas of Sion: Text and Translation* (Brookline, Mass.: Hellenic College Press, 1984), pp. 11, 105.

15. Geanakoplos, *Byzantium: Church, Society, and Civilization*, p. 430. George Pournaropoulos, "Medicine in Temples and Churches: Divine and Priestly Healing" (in Greek), in *Antidoron Pneumatikon*, pp. 417–25.

16. Ioannes N. Kardamitses, *The History of the Panhellenic Sacred Foundation of the Virgin of the Annunciation* (in Greek) (Athens: Ekdosis Hierou Hidrymatos, 1960), p. 25.

17. Telephone interview with Nicholas Soteropoulos, 9 September 1986.

18. Michael S. Rosco, "You Are the God Who Creates Miracles": The Story of Our Lady of Chicago" (Johnstown, Pa.: Carpatho-Russian Orthodox Greek Catholic Diocese, n.d.). See also Alexander Atty, "Our Lady of Chicago" and "A Pilgrimage to See the Weeping Icon," *Word* 31, no. 4 (1987).

19. Gregory (*PG* 66:740) is quoted in Gendle, "Role of the Byzantine Saint," p. 183. The document mentioning Stephen, *Epistula Luciani (Patrologia Latina*, ed. J. P. Migne, 221 vols. [Paris, 1844–64]), is quoted in E. D. Hunt, "The Traffic in Relics: Some Late Roman Evidence," in *Byzantine Saint*, ed. Hackel, p. 171. (*Patrologia Latina* is hereafter cited as *PL*.)

170 :   *Health and Medicine in the Eastern Orthodox Tradition*

20. "Saints Called Upon for Special Purposes," *Sacred Art Journal: Orthodox Liturgical Arts* 6, no. 3 (July–September 1985): 52–58.
21. *Menaion* for 1 November (unpublished St. Vladimir's Seminary translation).
22. *Menaion* for 22 December (unpublished St. Vladimir's Seminary translation).

Chapter 9/ Spiritual Healing: The Liturgy

1. Timothy (Kallistos) Ware, *The Orthodox Church* (Baltimore: Penguin Books, 1965), p. 269.
2. In addition to the shorter service book (Greek, *Mikron Euchologion;* Slavonic, *Trebnik*) used by the priest in his liturgical ministrations, the "Great Prayer Book" (*Mega Euchologion*) includes many services and prayers for specific situations.
3. The best treatment of the sacramental perspective of Eastern Orthodoxy is Alexander Schmemann, *For the Life of the World* (Crestwood, N.Y.: St. Vladimir's Seminary Press, 1982). A deeper treatment of the liturgical dimension of Orthodox life can be found in Schmemann, *Introduction to Liturgical Theology,* trans. Asheleigh E. Moorhouse (Portland, Maine: American Orthodox Press, 1966).
4. The translations from the baptismal service are from *Orthodox Prayer Book,* pp. 46–73 (slight modifications in the translation have been made).
5. The translation "a healing of sickness" (pp. 59–60) is incorrect. The Greek is *nosematon alexiterion.*
6. Translations of the Divine Liturgy and associated prayers are from *The Divine Liturgy: A New Translation by Members of the Faculty of Hellenic College/ Holy Cross Greek Orthodox School of Theology* (Brookline, Mass.: Holy Cross Orthodox Press, 1985).
7. *Byzantine Daily Worship: With Byzantine Breviary, the Three Liturgies, Propers of the Day and Various Offices,* ed. Joseph Raya and José de Vink (Allendale, N.J.: Alleluia Press, 1969), p. 333.
8. *Divine Prayers and Services of the Catholic Orthodox Church of Christ,* ed. Seraphim Nassar (Englewood, N.J.: Antiochian Orthodox Christian Archdiocese of North America, 1979), p. 105.
9. For the bibliographic notations to the patristic references in this paragraph, see *A Patristic Greek Lexicon,* ed. G. W. H. Lampe (Oxford: Clarendon Press, 1968), s.v. "*pharmakon, to.*"
10. For more about the sacrament of confession in the Orthodox tradition, see John Erickson, "Penitential Discipline in the Orthodox Canonical Tradition," *St. Vladimir's Theological Quarterly* 21 (1977): 200–201, from which this passage is quoted. See also Stanley S. Harakas, "Theology of the Sacrament of Holy Confession," *Greek Orthodox Theological Review* 19 (1974): 177–201, and "Theological Brief on the Forgiveness of Sins," in *Christian Theology: A Case Method Approach,* ed. Robert A. Evans and Thomas D. Parker (New York: Harper and Row, 1976).
11. Constantine Cavarnos, "The Role of Orthodox Monasticism in America," lecture given at the 50th Anniversary Celebration Intra-Orthodox Conference on Pas-

toral Praxis, Holy Cross Greek Orthodox School of Theology, Brookline, Mass., 25 September 1986. Quoted with permission.

12. "Commentary on the Gospel of Matthew," Homily 27, 2. *Nicene and Post-Nicene Fathers*, 2d ser. 10:185.

13. Michael B. Henning, *Marriage and the Christian Home* (Jordanville, N.Y.: Holy Trinity Monastery, 1976), pp. 30–31.

14. "The Service of the Small Paraklesis to the Most Holy Theotokos" (Brookline, Mass.: Holy Cross Orthodox Press, 1984).

15. Ibid., pp. 15, 21, 24, 25, 27, 34, 36.

16. Ibid., p. 15.

17. Ibid., p. 27.

18. Ibid., p. 29.

19. I have here followed the description of Chrestos M. Enisleides, *The Institution of Fasting: Faith and Life-style of the Church from an Orthodox Perspective* (in Greek) (Athens: Enoria Publications, 1959) chaps. 4–6.

20. Ibid., pp. 68–69.

21. Canon 69 of the Apostolic Canons. *The Rudder*, ed. Agapius and Nicodemus, trans. D. Cummings (Chicago: Orthodox Christian Education Society, 1957), p. 122. See also the commentary on this canon, pp. 125–27.

22. Enisleides, *Institution of Fasting*, p. 199.

23. *Orthodox Prayer Book*, p. 140.

24. See George C. Papademetriou, "Exorcism in the Orthodox Church," in *A Companion to the Greek Orthodox Church*, ed. Fotios K. Litsas (New York: Department of Communications of the Greek Orthodox Archdiocese, 1984), pp. 169–72.

25. For more on this ancient phenomenon, see Stanley S. Harakas, *The Orthodox Church: 455 Questions and Answers* (Minneapolis: Light and Life, 1987), questions 159, 160.

26. As examples, see Rev. Nicholas Paleologos, *Prayers for Eastern Orthodox Christians during Hospital Stay* (Privately published, n.d.); and *Meditation in Time of Sickness* (Boston: St. Andrew's Brotherhood, n.d.).

27. *Orthodox Prayer Book*, p. 18.

28. Ibid., pp. 24, 26–27.

29. Ibid., p. 21 (translation slightly revised). The Greek phrase retranslated is *phygadeueis tas nosous ton asthenounton.*

Chapter 10/ Spiritual Healing: Holy Unction

1. Alexander Schmemann may have done such spiritualizing in his *Sacraments and Orthodoxy* (New York: Herder and Herder, 1965), pp. 125–26.

2. See Elie Melia, "The Sacrament of the Anointing of the Sick: Its Historical Development and Current Practice," in *Temple of the Holy Spirit: Sickness and Death of the Christian in the Liturgy*, trans. Matthew J. O'Connell (New York: Pueblo, 1983), pp. 129–30; for the Talmudic reference (in the *Tractate Berakhot*) see p. 130.

3. Paul F. Palmer, *Sacraments and Forgiveness: History and Doctrinal Development of Penance, Extreme Unction and Indulgences* (Westminster, Md.: Newman Press, 1959), p. 277.

4. Dom Gregory Dix, ed., *The Treatise on the Apostolic Tradition of St. Hippolytus of Rome* 5.1–2 (London: S.P.C.K., 1937), p. 10. For a contemporary source, see the edition reissued with corrections, preface, and bibliography by Henry Chadwick (London: S.P.C.K., 1968).

5. *In Leviticum homilae* 2.4 (*PG* 12:418).

6. Aphaates, *Demonstrations*.

7. "Epistle 25.8: To Decentius."

8. *Prayer Book of Serapion* 2.10, Funk edition. For the texts and references to the passages in nn. 5–8, I am indebted to Palmer, *Sacraments and Forgiveness*, to which the reader is referred for additional information.

9. "All our evidence [indicating] that the top hospital administrators at Constantinople . . . were also medical doctors . . . comes from the twelfth century." Timothy S. Miller, *The Birth of the Hospital in the Byzantine Empire* (Baltimore: Johns Hopkins University Press, 1985), pp. 162–63.

10. Ibid., pp. 154–57.

11. Panagiotes N. Trembelas, *Mikron Euchologion* (in Greek), vol. 1, *The Services and Order of Engagement and Marriage, Unction, Ordination, and Baptism* (Athens, 1950), pp. 99–191, especially pp. 109–13. See also John M. Fountoulis, *The Liturgical Work of Symeon of Thessalonica* (in Greek) (Athens, 1966).

12. For the analysis of the material regarding the Scripture readings and the prayers, I am much indebted to Mark Sherman, who worked on these in a directed study of health and medicine in the Orthodox tradition in 1984–85 at Holy Cross Greek Orthodox School of Theology in Brookline, Massachusetts.

13. *Service Book of the Holy Orthodox-Catholic Apostolic Church*, pp. 340–41. I have revised the text significantly to reflect in contemporary English usage the precise meanings of Greek words directly related to health.

14. Ibid., p. 345. I have revised the text slightly to reflect contemporary English usage.

15. Anthony Coniaris, *Making God Real in the Orthodox Christian Home* (Minneapolis: Light and Life, 1977), pp. 131ff.

16. Henning, *Marriage and the Christian Home*, p. 31.

Chapter 11/ Passages: Beginnings

1. Scholars are able to estimate life expectancy of average citizens in ancient times on the basis of skeletal remains and sophisticated scientific dating procedures, using complex methods that coordinate numerous variables. See, for example, Jon Hendricks and C. Davis Hendricks, *Aging in Mass Society: Myths and Realities* (Cambridge, Mass.: Winthrop, 1977), pp. 32–33, esp. Fig. 2.2 and Table 2.1. For figures on the Byzantine period see Mary-Alice Talbot, "Old Age In Byzantium," *Byzantinische Zeitschrift* 77 (1984), pp. 265–66.

2. *Homilia in Psalmum 114*, 5 (*PG* 30:492–93); my translation.

3. Johannes Quasten, *Patrology*, vol. 3, *The Golden Age of Greek Patristic Literature from the Council of Nicea to the Council of Chalcedon* (Utrecht: Spectrum Publishers, 1966), p. 217.

4. *De Hominis Structura*, Oratio 1.17–18 (*PG* 30:25, 28); my translation.

5. Some representative writings of Lawrence Kohlberg are *The Philosophy of Moral Development: Moral Stages and the Idea of Justice* (San Francisco: Harper and Row, 1981); "Moral Stages and Moralization: A Cognitive Developmental Approach," in *Moral Development and Behavior*, ed. T. Licknon (New York: Holt, Rinehart and Winston, 1976); "Stages of Moral Development as a Basis for Moral Education" and "Educating for a Just Society: An Updated and Revised Statement," in *Moral Development, Moral Education, and Kohlberg: Basic Issues in Philosophy, Psychology, Religion, and Education*, ed. Brenda Muncey (Birmingham, Ala.: Religious Education Press, 1980).

6. James W. Fowler, *Stages of Faith: The Psychology of Human Development and the Quest for Meaning* (San Francisco: Harper and Row, 1981); *Becoming Adult, Becoming Christian: Adult Development and Christian Faith* (New York: Harper and Row, 1984).

7. Carol Gilligan, *In a Different Voice: Psychological Theory and Women's Development* (Cambridge, Mass.: Harvard University Press, 1982); "In a Different Voice: Women's Conceptions of Self and Morality," *Harvard Educational Review* 47 (1977); "Woman's Place in Man's Life Cycle," *Harvard Educational Review* 49 (1979).

8. John T. Chirban, *Human Growth and Faith: Intrinsic and Extrinsic Motivation in Human Development* (Washington, D.C.: University Press of America, 1981); "Developmental Stages in Eastern Orthodox Christianity," in *Transformations of Consciousness: Conventional and Contemplative Perspectives on Development*, ed. Ken Wilber et al. (Boston: New Science Library, 1986), chap. 9.

9. Gail Sheehy, *Passages* (New York: Bantam Press, 1977).

10. See, for example, Brenda Muncey, ed., *Moral Development, Moral Education, and Kohlberg: Basic Issues in Philosophy, Psychology, Religion, and Education* (Birmingham, Ala.: Religious Education Press, 1980); Gary L. Sapp, *Handbook of Moral Development* (Birmingham, Ala.: Religious Education Press, 1986).

11. See, for example, Donald M. Joy, *Moral Development Foundations: Judeo-Christian Alternatives to Piaget/Kohlberg* (Nashville: Abingdon Press, 1983).

12. An example of this approach for the Orthodox is found in Alexander Kazhdan and Giles Constable, *People and Power in Byzantium: An Introduction to Modern Byzantine Studies* (Washington, D.C.: Dumbarton Oaks Center for Byzantine Studies, 1982), pp. 62–63.

13. *Orthodox Prayer Book*, pp. 78, 82.

14. *Orthodox Prayer Book*, pp. 83–87.

15. Significantly, the original Greek text from the *Mega Euchologion* (reprinted in the common *Priest's Prayer Book* in Greek) titles this collection of prayers "On the First Day after a Woman Has Given Birth to a Child." However, in Vaporis's bilingual edition of the *Prayer Book*, the title is "Prayers on the Birth of a Child," reflecting, unconsciously perhaps, the changes forced on the clergy by hospital practice, communication delays, and so on.

16. *Orthodox Prayer Book*, pp. 32–36.

17. *Orthodox Prayer Book*, p. 39.

18. The paragraphs dealing with the Service of the Churching are based in part on my answer given in the "Religious Question Box" column of the nationally circulated Greek-American weekly *The Hellenic Chronicle* (12 June 1986) in response to the question "Why is it in our Church a woman who has just given birth has to wait forty days to attend Church services?"

19. Alcibiadis C. Calivas, "The Sacramental Life of the Orthodox Church," in *A Companion to the Greek Orthodox Church*, ed. Fotios K. Litsas (New York: Department of Communications of the Greek Orthodox Archdiocese of North and South America, 1984), p. 36. For more on infant baptism from an Orthodox perspective see Jordan Bajis, *Infant Baptism* (New York: Department of Communications of the Greek Orthodox Archdiocese of North and South America, 1983).

20. Calivas, "Sacramental Life," p. 37.

21. For a fuller, more balanced discussion of the Eucharist, see Calivas, "Sacramental Life," pp. 40–46.

Chapter 12/ Passages toward Maturation

1. Quoted in *The Christian Way of Life*, ed. Francis X. Murphy (Wilmington, Del.: Michael Glazier, 1986), p. 35.

2. See Cecil John Cadoux, *The Early Church and the World* (Edinburgh: T. and T. Clark, 1955), p. 445.

3. From the commentary on canon 60 of the Sixth Ecumenical Council. *Rudder*, p. 336. See pp. 335–38 for the full discussion.

4. M. L. W. Laistner, *Christianity and Pagan Culture in the Later Roman Empire: Together with an English Translation of John Chrysostom's "Address on Vainglory and the Right Way for Parents to Bring Up Their Children"* (Ithaca, N.Y.: Cornell University Press, 1951).

5. Quasten, *Patrology* 3:214.

6. For example, the percentage of college-educated Greek Orthodox Christians in the United States is one of the highest in the nation. "According to the 1970 census, Greek American men and women were 70 percent more likely to have completed college than the native white population." Charles C. Moskos, Jr., *Greek Americans: Struggle and Success* (Englewood Cliffs, N.J.: Prentice-Hall, 1980), pp. 111–12.

7. For a description of the varied evaluations of sex in the Orthodox tradition see Joseph Allen, "Practical Issues of Sexuality," *St. Vladimir's Theological Quarterly* 27, no. 1 (1983): 44–45. Sexuality and sex in marriage according to patristic thought and church teaching are also discussed in Demetrios J. Constantelos, *Marriage, Sexuality and Celibacy: A Greek Orthodox Perspective* (Minneapolis: Light and Life, 1975), pp. 18–43.

8. Few realize that in the life of the early church, the legitimacy and appropriateness of celibate living had to be defended and supported not only within the church but in the larger society. There were, for example, laws against those who were unmarried and did not procreate new citizens for the empire. They were

changed only by imperial decree in 320. See Rowan A. Greer, *Broken Lights and Mended Lives: Theology and Common Life in the Early Church* (University Park: Pennsylvania State University Press, 1986), p. 107.

9. In his admirable study of the marriage service, "Toward a Theology of Marriage in the Orthodox Church," Theodore Stylianopoulos says, "I tend by choice to anchor myself on St. John Chrysostom's thoroughly positive understanding of marriage rather than Symeon of Thessalonike's perception of marriage as a concession to human weakness by God's mercy." *Greek Orthodox Theological Review* 22, no. 3 (1977): 249–83.

10. A survey of contemporary Orthodox literature on marriage and the family supports this statement. Some representative titles are Vladimir Berzonsky, *The Gift of Love* (Crestwood, N.Y.: St. Vladimir's Seminary Press, 1985); Anthony Coniaris, *Getting Ready for Marriage in the Orthodox Church* (Minneapolis: Light and Life, 1972); George Nicozisin, *Your Marriage in the Orthodox Church* (St. Louis: privately published, 1982).

11. 1 Timothy 3.

12. *Rudder*, p. 524. See also Apostolic Canon 5 and canons 6 and 33 of Carthage.

13. Characteristic is canon 33 of the Council of Elvira, Spain, held about the year 306: "Bishops, presbyters, deacons, and others with a position in the ministry are to abstain completely from sexual intercourse with their wives and from the procreation of children. If anyone disobeys, he shall be removed from clerical office." Jan L. Womer, trans. and ed., *Morality and Ethics in Early Christianity* (Philadelphia: Fortress Press, 1987), p. 78. It was not for another four or five centuries that this view became fully dominant in the Western part of the church.

14. Ibid., p. 305.

15. Ibid., pp. 305–6. The "injunction handed down by the Apostles" refers to the Pauline teaching in 1 Corinthians 7:1–7 that married couples may, by agreement, avoid sexual relations for designated periods of time for the sake of prayer and devotion but should not do so permanently. The reference to the Council of Carthage, held in 418, is to canons 3 and 4 which address the question of clergy who are prohibited from sexual relations when they are to serve the altar.

16. Paul Evdokimoff, *The Struggle with God*, trans. Sister Gertrude, S.P. (Glen Rock, N.J.: Paulist Press, 1966), p. 73.

17. "Be fruitful and multiply" (Genesis 1:27); "It is not good that man should be alone; I will make him a helper fit for him" (Genesis 2:18).

18. "The Grace of the Holy Spirit is bestowed to sanctify the union of man and wife, and to enable them to attain the end which marriage has in view." Constantine Dyobouniotes, quoted in Frank Gavin, *Some Aspects of Contemporary Greek Orthodox Thought* (London: Society for Promoting Christian Knowledge, 1936), p. 378.

19. Michael Kardamakis, *Love and Marriage* (in Greek) (Athens: Akritas Publications, 1981), p. 15 (my translation; emphasis in original).

20. For the reasons see John Meyendorff, *Marriage: An Orthodox Perspective* (Crestwood, N.Y.: St. Vladimir's Seminary Press, 1970), pp. 27–32.

21. The Service of the Promise and the Service of Marriage are found in *Orthodox Prayer Book*, pp. 75–76, 87. Stylianopoulos, "Toward a Theology of Marriage,"

gives a good summary of the varied meanings given to the crowns from the time of St. John Chrysostom (fourth century), p. 261, n. 38.

22. Stanley S. Harakas, "The Orthodox Church," in *Ecumenical and Pastoral Guidelines and Pastoral Directives on Christian Marriage* (Boston: Whittemore, n.d.). Also published as *Guidelines for Marriage in the Orthodox Church* (Minneapolis: Light and Life, n.d.).

23. *Documents of the Orthodox Church in America: Marriage* (Orthodox Church in America, n.d.), p. 15. In the churches of the Greek tradition a formal divorce proceeding is held in an ecclesiastical court.

24. According to an encyclical letter of 21 November 1973 (Protocol No. 206A) of the Greek Orthodox Archdiocese of North and South America, divorces may be granted by ecclesiastical courts on the basis of the following ten criteria: (a) when the marriage was begun through violence or force, or when these are part of the ongoing marital relationship; (b) if one of the spouses is an adulterer; (c) when mental illness is judged incurable in one of the spouses, or if a venereal disease existed before marriage and was not disclosed prior to the marriage; (d) when one of the spouses is shown to have sought the death of the other; (e) when one of the spouses is sentenced to prison for a period of more than seven years; (f) when, without the agreement of the other spouse, a marriage partner abandons bed and board for a period of more than three years; (g) when the abandonment takes place for any reason other than mental illness; (h) when the husband forces his wife into adulterous relations or prostitution; (i) when the sexual relations of the couple are not naturally fulfilled, or when reasons exist that do not allow natural sexual relations to take place; (j) when behaviors (e.g., alcoholism, compulsive gambling) cause severe and unresolved economic problems.

25. Some have called for a change in this practice (see Demetrios J. Constantelos, *Marriage, Sexuality and Celibacy*), but it has not been widely debated.

26. An interesting and practical attempt at rehabilitating the consecrated single life in our day in the Roman Catholic Church is Benedict J. Groeschel's *Courage to Be Chaste* (New York: Paulist Press, 1985).

Chapter 13/ Maturity and Development

1. Harakas, *Toward Transfigured Life*, esp. chaps. 2 and 3.

2. For a popular short life of St. Katherine, see George Poulos, *Orthodox Saints* (Brookline, Mass.: Holy Cross Orthodox Press, 1976), 1:179–80.

3. For the life of St. Ephrosynos the Cook (c. 1750), ibid., 1:133–34. For an example of the life of a neomartyr, see the story of St. Akilina (d. 1764), ibid., 1:137–38.

4. Christophoros Stavropoulos, *Partakers of Divine Nature* trans. Stanley S. Harakas (Minneapolis: Light and Life, 1976), pp. 37–38.

5. Panagiotes K. Chrestou, *Partakers of God* (Brookline, Mass.: Holy Cross Orthodox Press, 1984); Stanley S. Harakas, *Toward Transfigured Life*, chap. 7; Vladimir Lossky, *In the Image and Likeness of God*, ed. John H. Erickson and Thomas E. Bird (Crestwood, N.Y.: St. Vladimir's Seminary Press, 1974); A. J. Philippou, ed., *Orthodoxy: Life and Freedom* (Oxford: Studion Publications, 1973);

Robert Slesinski, *Pavel Florensky: A Metaphysics of Love* (Crestwood, N.Y.: St. Vladimir's Seminary Press, 1984); Christos Yannaras, *The Freedom of Morality* (Crestwood, N.Y.: St. Vladimir's Seminary Press, 1984); John D. Zizioulas, *Being As Communion: Studies in Personhood and the Church* (Crestwood, N.Y.: St. Vladimir's Seminary Press, 1985).

6. Fowler, *Becoming Adult, Becoming Christian*, p. 141.

7. In Orthodox theology the term *synergy*, while referring to both God and humans, focuses on human cooperation with God (who is the chief agent of our salvation) rather than on God's cooperation with us.

8. That this, too, is part of the living tradition of the early church has been noted by Greer, in *Broken Lights and Mended Lives*, pp. 7–16.

9. For a vigorous and critical expression of this reality see Eva C. Topping, "Patriarchal Prejudice and Pride in Greek Christianity: Some Notes on Origins," *Journal of Modern Greek Studies* 1, no. 1 (1983): 7–17. For a positive statement of the same assessment, see Topping's "Thekla the Nun: In Praise of Women," *Greek Orthodox Theological Review* 25 (1980): 353–70.

10. Kyriaki FitzGerald, "The Ministry of Women in the Orthodox Church: Some Theological Presuppositions," *Journal of Ecumenical Studies* 20, no. 4 (Fall 1983): 558–75, and "The Characteristics and Nature of the Order of the Deaconess," in *Women and the Priesthood*, ed. Thomas Hopko (Crestwood, N.Y.: St. Vladimir's Seminary Press, 1983), pp. 75–96.

11. Bk. 1, chap. 4.

12. "On the Death of His Father," Oration 18. *Nicene and Post-Nicene Fathers*, 2d ser. 7:257.

13. The balanced work of the following Orthodox women theologians both explain and challenges the status of women in the Orthodox church: Deborah Belonick, *Feminism in Christianity: An Orthodox Christian Response* (Crestwood, N.Y.: Orthodox Church in America, 1981); FitzGerald, "Ministry of Women in the Orthodox Church"; Kyriaki FitzGerald, "Orthodox Women and Pastoral Praxis: Observation and Concerns for the Church in America," in *Orthodox Perspectives on Pastoral Praxis*, ed. Theodore Stylianopoulos, 101–26 (Brookline, Mass.: Holy Cross Orthodox Press, 1988); and *Orthodox Women: Their Role and Participation in the Orthodox Church*, ed. Constance Tarasar and Irina Kirillva (Geneva: World Council of Churches, 1977).

14. The preceding few paragraphs are a revision of a portion of the first part of Stanley S. Harakas, "The Moral Dimension of Christian Man-Woman Relationships," *Orthodox Observer* 36 (October 1970): 11.

15. One of the earliest modern treatments of bioethical issues from an Orthodox perspective is Stanley S. Harakas, "Eastern Orthodox Christianity," *Encyclopedia of Bioethics*, ed. Warren T. Reich (Washington, D.C.: Georgetown University Press, 1978), 1:347–55. The article was republished in a slightly modified form as a pamphlet: *For the Health of Body and Soul: An Eastern Orthodox Introduction to Bioethics* (Brookline, Mass.: Holy Cross Orthodox Press, 1980).

16. *Orthodox Prayer Book*, pp. 91, 96.

17. See Harakas, *Toward Transfigured Life*, chap. 4.

18. For more development of this topic from an Orthodox ethical perspective see Harakas, *For the Health of Body and Soul*, pp. 37–40, and Stanley S. Harakas,

Contemporary Moral Issues Facing the Orthodox Christian (Minneapolis: Light and Life, 1982), secs. 18–20, 24–26, 29. More generally, see Constantelos, *Marriage, Sexuality and Celibacy*, and Meyendorff, *Marriage: An Orthodox Perspective*.

19. On abortion, see Harakas, *For the Health of Body and Soul*, pp. 29–30, and Harakas, *Contemporary Moral Issues*, secs. 22, 36.

20. There are many treatments of the subject by Orthodox theologians. For brief descriptions of the debate within Orthodox Christianity on contraception with reference as well to population issues see Harakas, *For the Health of Body and Soul*, pp. 40–44, and Harakas, *Contemporary Moral Issues*, sec. 21.

21. Gabriel Dionysiatou, *Malthusianism: The Crime of Genocide* (in Greek) (Volos: Holy Mountain Library, 1954); Athenagoras Kokkinakis, *Parents and Priests as Servants of Redemption* (New York: Morehouse-Gorham, 1985), pp. 56–60; Serapheim Papacostas, *The Question of the Procreation of Children: The Demographic Problem from a Christian Viewpoint* (in Greek) (Athens: Zoe Publications, 1933, 1947).

22. Nearly all the American Orthodox writers on the topic of marriage noted previously hold to this view. However, the best exposition is in Chrysostom Zafires, "The Morality of Contraception: An Eastern Orthodox Opinion," *Journal of Ecumenical Studies* 11 (1974): 33–54. See also Nicon D. Patrinacos, *The Orthodox Church on Birth Control* (Garwood, N.J.: Graphic Arts Press, 1975).

23. Stanley S. Harakas, "Christian Faith Concerning Creation and Biology." *La Théologie dans L'Eglise et dans le Monde* (Geneva: Editions du Centre Orthodoxe du Patriarchat Oecouménique, 1984), secs. 1, 2.

24. Canons 21, 23, and 24 of the Apostolic Canons, and canon 1 of the First Ecumenical Council. *Rudder*, pp. 33–35, 163.

25. Harakas, *For the Health of Body and Soul*, pp. 44ff.

26. Harakas, *For the Health of Body and Soul*, pp. 44–46, and Harakas, *Contemporary Moral Issues*, sec. 23.

27. Harakas, *For the Health of Body and Soul*, p. 47.

28. Some predominantly Eastern Orthodox populations do have relatively widespread occurrences of genetically derived diseases, for example, thalassemia, mentioned in Chapter 7. See Stanley S. Harakas, "Thalassemia: A Theological Perspective," chap. 6 of *Thalassemia: An Interdisciplinary Approach*, ed. Chirban.

29. The participants, in order of their offices mentioned in the text, were Dr. George J. Pazin of the University of Pittsburgh School of Medicine, Chaplain Peter Poulos of the Brooklyn Methodist Hospital, Dr. Chirban of OCAMPR, Rev. Stanley S. Harakas of Holy Cross Greek Orthodox School of Theology, Evi Hatziandreu of the Department of Health and Human Services, and Rev. Miltiades Efthimiou of the Greek Orthodox Archdiocese Department of Church and Society.

Chapter 14/ "Trampling on Death"

1. William E. Phipps, *Death: Confronting the Reality* (Atlanta: John Knox Press, 1987), pp. iv, v.

2. Quoted by Anne Fremantle, *New York Times Book Review*, 28 September, 1958. In *The Great Quotations*, ed. George Seldes (New York, Pocket Books, 1967), p. 255.

3. *Orthodox Prayer Book*, p. 107.

4. James P. Carse, *Death and Existence: A Conceptual History of Human Mortality* (New York: John Wiley and Sons, 1980). This paragraph restates in summary form the outline of the contents of Carse's volume.

5. Besides Carse, *Death and Existence*, see, for example, Philippe Ariès, *Western Attitudes toward Death: From the Middle Ages to the Present* (Baltimore: Johns Hopkins University Press, 1974); Panos D. Bardis, *History of Thanatology: Philosophical, Religious, and Sociological Ideas Concerning Death from Primitive Times to the Present* (Washington, D.C.: University Press of America, 1981); Jacques Choron, *Death and Western Thought* (New York: Collier Books, 1963); Norbert Greinacher and Alois Muller, eds., *The Experience of Dying* (New York: Herder and Herder, 1974); Robert Kastenbaum and Ruth Aisenberg, *The Psychology of Death* (New York: Springer, 1972); Elisabeth Kübler-Ross, *On Death and Dying* (New York: Macmillan, 1969); Kübler-Ross, *Death: The Final Stage of Growth* (Englewood Cliffs, N.J.: Prentice-Hall, 1975); F. Warren Shibles, *Death: An Interdisciplinary Analysis* (Whitewater, Wis.: Language Press, 1974); Edwin S. Shneidman, ed., *Death: Current Perspectives* (New York: Jason Aronson, 1976).

6. Some representative books in reference to Orthodox thought and life are Constantine Callinicos, *Beyond the Grave: An Orthodox Theology of Eschatology*, trans. George Dimopoulos and Leslie Jerome Newville (Scranton, Pa.: Christian Orthodox Editions, 1969); Loring M. Danforth, *The Death Rituals of Rural Greece* (Princeton, N.J.: Princeton University Press, 1982); Philotheos Faros, *Penthos [Grief]: An Orthodox, Laographic and Psychological Perspective* (in Greek) (Athens: Akritas Publications, 1981); Lazar Puhalo, *The Soul, The Body and Death* (Chilliwack, British Columbia: Synaxis Press, 1985); Seraphim Rose, *The Soul After Death* (Platina, Calif.: Saint Herman of Alaska Brotherhood, 1980); Nicholas P. Vasiliades, *The Mystery of Death* (in Greek) (Athens: Soter Brotherhood Publications, 1980).

7. Epicurus, "Letter to Menoeceus," *The Philosophy of Epicurus*, ed. G. Strodach (Chicago: Northwestern University Press, 1963), pp. 178–95.

8. Harakas, *Contemporary Moral Issues*, p. 168.

9. Mary Warnock, *Existentialist Ethics* (New York: St. Martin's Press, 1967), p. 26.

10. Harakas, *Toward Transfigured Life*, pp. 60–61.

11. Elisabeth Kübler-Ross, *On Death and Dying*.

12. Kübler-Ross, *Death: The Final Stage of Growth*, pp. 164, 166.

13. For two thorough treatments comparing this classical view with other teachings on the doctrine of the atonement, see Gustaf Aulén, *Christus Victor: An Historical Study of the Three Main Types of the Idea of the Atonement*, trans. A. G. Hebert (London: S.P.C.K., 1965), and Jaroslav Pelikan, *The Shape of Death: Life, Death, and Immortality in the Early Fathers* (New York: Abingdon Press, 1961).

14. Theodore of Mopsuestia (350–428), *Catechetical Homilies* 14.5. Quoted in Joanne E. McWilliam Dewart, *Death and Resurrection*, vol. 22 of the Message of the Fathers of the Church series (Wilmington, Del.: Michael Glazier, 1986), p. 161.

15. Phipps, *Death*, pp. 129–30.

16. *Book of Divine Prayers and Services of the Catholic Orthodox Church of Christ*, comp. Seraphim Nassar (New York: Blackshaw Press, 1938), pp. 137–38.

17. Constantine Callinicos gives a full description of Orthodox theological perspectives on death in *Beyond the Grave: An Orthodox Theology of Eschatology*. For liturgical and ritual treatment of death in Byzantium, see Dorothy Abrahamse, "Rituals of Death in the Middle Byzantine Period," *Greek Orthodox Theological Review* 29, no. 2 (1984): 125.

18. Danforth, *Death Rituals of Rural Greece*, pp. 12–20, 71ff.

19. The rites for the dead vary slightly among the various Orthodox ecclesiastical jurisdictions. I am describing here general practice in the Greek Orthodox Archdiocese of North and South America. See *Orthodox Prayer Book*, pp. 97–132.

20. For a full description, see James Kyriakakis, "Byzantine Burial Customs: Care of the Deceased from Death to the Prothesis," *Greek Orthodox Theological Review* 19, no. 1 (1974): 37–72.

21. Constantine Callinicos, *The Christian Temple and the Services Conducted in It* (in Greek) (Athens: Ekthesis Christianikou Bibliou, 1958), pp. 594–95.

22. The sixth and eighth books of the *Apostolic Constitutions*, written in the latter half of the fourth century, record descriptions of such a service and associated practices. See Callinicos, *Christian Temple*, pp. 594–95, and Pangagiotes Trembelas, *Liturgical Types of Egypt and the East: A Contribution to the History of Christian Worship* (in Greek) (Athens: Apostolic Diakonia Press, 1961), pp. 318–19.

23. *Dionysius the Pseudo-Areopagite*, trans. Thomas L. Campbell (Washington, D.C.: University Press of America, 1981), pp. 79–91.

24. Callinicos, *Christian Temple*, pp. 596–97.

25. *Threskeytike kai Ethike Enkyklopaideia* 9:383–84, s.v. Nekrosimos Akolouthia, Kedeia (Funeral Service)

26. *Threskeytike kai Ethike Enkyklopaideia* 9: 385.

27. Paul J. Fedwick, "Death and Dying in the Byzantine Liturgical Tradition," *Eastern Churches Review* 8, no. 2 (1976): 152–61.

28. Boris Bobrinskoy, "Old Age and Death: Tragedy or Blessing," *St. Vladimir's Theological Quarterly* 28, no. 4 (1984): 244.

29. Vasiliades, *Mystery of Death*, p. 339.

30. *Greek Orthodox Theological Review* 29, no. 2 (1984): 201.

31. *To Penthos [Grief]: An Orthodox, Laographic and Psychological Perspective* (in Greek) (Athens: Akritas Publications, 1981). See also Joseph J. Allen, "The Orthodox Pastor and the Dying," *St. Vladimir's Theological Quarterly* 23, no. 1 (1979): 23–40. Allen does not deal extensively with the service. He does, however, note the service's emphasis on the reality of death and its "reconstructive" power.

32. Faros, *Penthos*, pp. 344–45, 362–65.

33. Ibid., pp. 141–50, 185–87, 252–55.

34. Ibid., pp. 157ff.

35. For fuller statements on these and other moral issues see three works by Stanley S. Harakas: *Contemporary Moral Issues, For the Health of Body and Soul*, and *Let Mercy Abound: Social Concern in the Greek Orthodox Church* (Brookline, Mass.: Holy Cross Orthodox Press, 1983).

36. See Harakas, *Let Mercy Abound,* for several such statements: Twentieth Clergy-Laity Congress (1970), pp. 128–29, and Twenty-third Clergy-Laity Congress (1976), pp. 144–45.

37. For Orthodox statements on euthanasia, see the articles by Thomas Hopko and Stanley Harakas in *Euthanasia And Religion: A Survey of the Attitudes of World Religions to the Right-To-Die,* ed. Gerald A. Larue (Los Angeles: Hemlock Society, 1985), pp. 45–57.

Index